ONE
MAN'S
FOOD...

ONE MAN'S FOOD

... is someone else's poison

DR. JAMES D'ADAMO
with ALLAN RICHARDS

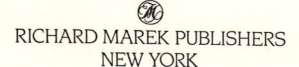

RICHARD MAREK PUBLISHERS
NEW YORK

Library of Congress Cataloging in Publication Data

D'Adamo, James L
    One man's food—is someone else's poison.

    Bibliography: p.
    Includes index.
    1. Diet. 2. Nutrition. 3. Diet therapy.
4. Blood groups—ABO system. 5. Naturopathy.
I. Richards, Allan, joint author. II. Title.
RA784.D32   615.8'54   80-20019
ISBN 0-399-90092-6

To Dr. L. J. B. Cardinal N.D., D.N.B., M.D., Chairman of the National Board of Naturopathic. Examiners, whose many years of devotion, toil, and sacrifice have greatly enriched the profession of Naturopathy.

Contents

Contents

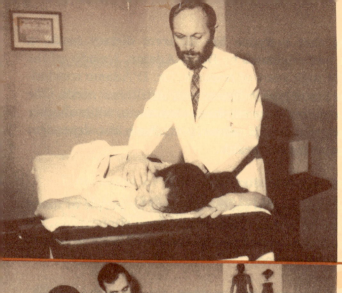

• Massage

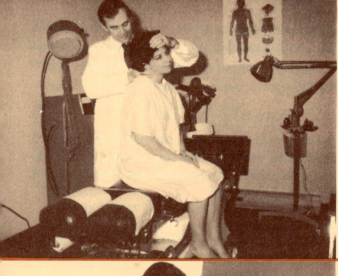

• Chiropractic treatment

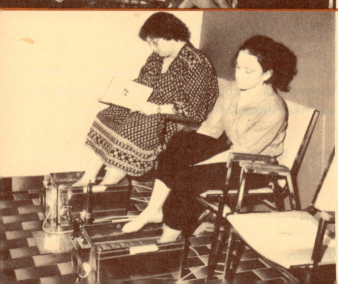

• Foot bath

> In man's endeavor to strive forward, he should never lose sight of his origin, which lies in nature. He should always know that nature, being the creator of life, is best equipped to maintain the life it created.
>
> Dr. James L. D'Adamo

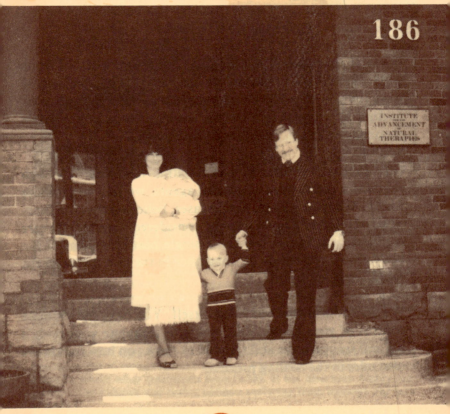

INSTITUTE
for the
ADVANCEMENT
of
NATURAL THERAPIES

- 186 St. George Street
Toronto, Canada M5R 2N3
(416) 968-0496

- 1472 Bay Ridge Parkway
Brooklyn, N.Y. 11228, U.S.A.
(212) 236-5059

- Montego Bay, Jamaica
West Indies

"One should not eat according to the taste buds. Instead, the foods to be consumed should be chosen wisely with the understanding as to which foods will give strength to the individual body."

—Jewish Law

ONE MAN'S FOOD...

PREFACE

I first heard about Dr. D'Adamo five years ago, the day I was introduced to my wife-to-be, Ingrid. We were fellow guests at a country cottage in upstate New York and our hostess had been extravagant in her praise of her doctor and the remarkable diet he had created for her, based on—of all things—her blood type. Since she had been on the regimen, she told us, she had lost weight, she felt younger, her complexion had become smoother and she had boundless energy—important benefits indeed to one who, like Ingrid, was a fashion model.

"Another diet," I thought, "ho hum." Ingrid, however, was immediately interested. Having been a vegetarian for ten years under the care of a London nutritionist, she was eager to receive continued guidance in her new home, New York. Several weeks later, after Ingrid and I were married, she had her first appointment with Dr. D'Adamo.

Ingrid and I had many things to learn about each other, and at first I feared I'd married a health fanatic since she thought nothing of traveling an hour-and-a-half by subway from our Manhattan apartment to Dr. D'Adamo's office in Brooklyn. When she returned from her appointment, she was very excited.

"He diagnoses by looking into your eyes," she exclaimed. "You fill out a form about your illnesses but without ever looking at it, he tells you your entire medical history. Then, he determines whether you should eat meat or be a vegetarian, and what vitamins and herbs to take by your blood type. Darling, I think *you* should see him."

Although Ingrid had appeared to be the picture of health while on her vegetarian regimen, with lovely skin, clear bright eyes and an effervescent personality, Dr. D'Adamo discovered that she was anemic, that she had weakened her left ovary and unbalanced her hormonal system from a lack of protein, and that she had a weakened heart valve from a childhood illness. Because her blood type was O, he prescribed a high animal-protein diet, with a daily allowance of chicken, fish, liver or veal. Because Ingrid had been a vegetarian for so long, this kind of diet was unappealing at first. However, she followed it and after one month on the new diet, she had a resurgence of energy, and no longer required her afternoon naps.

In the past I had experimented with various diets: vegetarian, fruit and macrobiotics. None of them ever seemed right for me: I always felt faint and enervated after being on them for a while. My only current physical discomforts were pains in my fingers, which I attributed to practicing the piano, and a few boils on my shoulders, which I assumed were caused by the oil from my then-long hair. Though I was interested in obtaining professional nutritional guidance and had acknowledged Ingrid's new vitality, I was skeptical that a legitimate doctor could diagnose your medical history through your eyes or design an individualized diet by your blood type. (I was particularly suspicious because at that time quack healers, amateur psychics, spiritual mountebanks—anyone with a program for salvation—were much in vogue.)

I told Ingrid I would try her diet. "No, not mine," she insisted, "because we are individuals with different needs; what may be good for my body may not be good for yours." It seemed like good common sense, and for the sake of marital harmony, I agreed to see the doctor. However, I knew it would be nearly impossible to arrange an appointment since we were leaving for California for six months, and I had heard that there was a long list of people waiting to see him. As luck (or fate) would have it, three days before we were to leave Dr. D'Adamo's nurse called. A patient had cancelled his appointment, would I like it? Joking that this would be her wedding present to me, Ingrid hustled me onto the subway to Bay Ridge, Brooklyn, and Dr. D'Adamo's office.

Needless to say, I had many preconceptions. I imagined his office to be a meeting place for all sorts of weird-looking health faddists. Many people I knew involved in offbeat diets looked the same: blond matured versions of the sixties San Francisco hippie scene flashing neon smiles. I was surprised, and somewhat

2

reassured, when I encountered a broad cross section of people in the waiting room: conservatively dressed professional types, old folks, mothers with babies, a rabbinical student and one representative of the counterculture. Times have changed, I thought.

While waiting to see Dr. D'Adamo, I was given the medical-history questionnaire that Ingrid had told me about. I noted the current pains in my fingers, such childhood illnesses as mumps and measles, a case of sinusitis and a teenage back injury. For family history, I noted that my maternal grandmother had suffered with severe arthritis in her hands and feet. I omitted reference to the boils on my shoulders; I wanted to see if the doctor would detect them in his diagnosis.

Before my examination began, Dr. D'Adamo introduced himself and explained that I might be unfamiliar with his methods of diagnosis and treatment. He said he would examine me with a method called iridology, diagnosis through observation of the iris of the eye. Through a complex neurological arrangement involving the cerebro-optic nerve, the iris acted as a physiological mirror of the body, he explained.

He also explained that the diet he would prepare for me would be based on the iridological findings and upon my blood type. He told me that he had found that a person's nutritional regimen could be determined by his blood type, A, O, B or AB. He asked me not to be hasty in my judgment of him, and advised me rather matter-of-factly, that if I followed his suggestions my body would be strengthened and any discomforts or abnormalities would be healed.

Without reviewing my medical history form, he commenced the examination (indeed, as Ingrid had said, he never did refer to the form). He rolled up my sleeve, took my blood pressure. Normal. He felt my pulse, while closing his eyes and, as if listening deep into my body with his fingertips, murmured, "Low body vitality, poor digestion." Next he raised his ophthalmoscope to my right eye and then my left. Among the things he observed were, "Mucus congestion in your lungs, a sluggish liver, weakened kidneys and adrenal glands. Do you

3

have pains in your hands?" he asked suddenly. "You're not getting enough sleep," he continued, "and your nervous system is badly stressed."

I was momentarily impressed; and quite honestly frightened by what I heard. Then I reminded myself that it was impossible to detect such things by looking into the eyes. Anyway it was such a general analysis. Who does get enough sleep? Who isn't anxious and stressed? But he did ask about pains in my hands. . . .

While I was assimilating what he said, Dr. D'Adamo gently pricked my finger and took a blood smear. He quickly analyzed it, then said, "You're a type B; come on into my office, let's get you fixed up with a diet."

Then I remembered he hadn't said anything about the boils on my shoulders, and, as if calling a bluff in a poker game, I mentioned this to him.

"You also have some scabs on your scalp, and some irritations on your thighs," he replied with a warm smile. "It's your liver. It's not cleaning your body efficiently; the wastes are seeping through your skin, causing eruptions. Don't worry about it, we'll clear it up in a couple of weeks." I was beginning to be less skeptical.

We passed the next hour in his office, preparing my diet. Because I had type B blood, he said that I would require a mixed vegetarian and animal-protein diet. He suggested I eat chicken, fish or veal three or four times a week, the other days eating grain such as brown rice, millet or buckwheat. I could have such fruits as grapefruit and cantaloupe, which would help purify my blood, but no oranges and tangerines, which are highly acidic and would irritate my weakened kidneys. He recommended that I reduce dairy products, eat only four eggs a week, and cheese and yogurt three times a week, because I already had an accumulation of mucus in my chest. Dairy products, he explained, were notorious mucus producers. Vegetables, condiments, breads, cereals, juices and vitamins were all likewise carefully prescribed according to my condition. I was also asked to reduce my intake of wine to once a week because my liver needed time to be cleansed and healed.

During the time I spent with Dr. D'Adamo, I began to understand Ingrid's words, "What may be good for my body may not be good for yours." Before my appointment ended, he encouraged me to question him.

"How long do I have to stay on the diet?" I asked.

"That's hard to say; each person responds differently. It depends on how quickly your body rebuilds itself, and how well you stay on the diet."

"Why can Ingrid have tomatoes while I can't?"

"They're too acidic for your body in its current state."

"Will I ever be able to eat them?"

"Yes, when your organs are cleansed and regenerated and the acidity no longer irritates their tissue."

As we parted, he told me to call him anytime if I had further questions. Then he said he didn't want to see me again for eight months!

I was impressed with the amount of time he spent with me (over two hours); his precision in selecting foods for my body; his patience in answering my questions; his concern that I felt comfortable with my diet (when I gibed at his recommendation that I reduce my consumption of eggs he replied, "Okay, if that's going to be a problem for you, have six or seven a week, but it would be better if you could cut down").

I was particularly surprised when he said he didn't want to see me on a regular basis. What doctor doesn't want to see patients every so often? He explained: "Deep healing takes time. You won't need a change in your diet for a while; besides, it would only be a unnecessary expense for you to see me again soon."

When I left his office, I felt "right" about Dr. D'Adamo and my diet. When something feels right, I don't think about doing it, I do it! After only two weeks on the regimen, like Ingrid, I, too, experienced a resurgence of energy—and the boils on my shoulders disappeared! During the six months Ingrid and I were in California, we stuck pretty much to our diets, only occasionally having a verboten piece of cheesecake. When we were rediagnosed upon returning to New York, Ingrid was no longer anemic, her ovary was again functioning normally and her heart valve had been strengthened. My digestion had been much improved, and though my liver had not yet fully regenerated, my scalp, thighs and shoulders were smooth and free of any blemishes.

In the five following years under Dr. D'Adamo's guidance, my body has continued to feel stronger and healthier, and I look much younger. At thirty, people tell me I look twenty. In contrast, when I was twenty-five, I had circles under my eyes and my skin was sallow and people mistook me for a thirty-five-year-old. I have had only two colds during this time, which is a dramatic triumph for me because before the diet I'd been resigned to having several colds a year and an annual bout of flu.

Am I still on his diet? Yes and no. I no longer think of myself as following a dietary regimen. It has become a way of life: eating foods that are harmonious and beneficial to my body's own individual needs.

I am frequently asked: "Who is Dr. D'Adamo? What is he like?" Briefly, I can say that in a time when medical doctors have become more and more specialized and detached from their patients, Dr. D'Adamo relates on a one-to-one basis; he gives each person the time and respect required to effect a total healing of his body. He is a gentle man, but not meek. He has treated many well-known and well-to-do people, yet he seems to shun celebrities and the limelight.

Dr. D'Adamo is a Diplomate in Naturopathy (the highest honor awarded a Naturopath, a physician who heals using only natural therapeutics) from the National Board of Naturopathic Examiners, the oldest examining board in the United States in any medical or healing art. In addition, he has increased his knowledge of dietetics, herbal remedies and other healing techniques by exhaustive studies at many of the finest health clinics

6

Preface

and offices in Switzerland, Germany, Norway, France, Austria and England.

He has been the Vice-President of the Naturopathic Association of Physicians of America, the President of the Naturopathic Society of New York, and the Liaison Officer representing the United States at the International Naturopathic Physicians Organization. His selfless efforts to establish Naturopathy as an alternative to conventional medicine has made him a symbol of the growing Naturopathic movement in America.

In the time I have known Dr. D'Adamo, I have never seen him rest; he has indefatigable energy. When not attending his patients, he is lecturing throughout America and Canada, teaching natural healing in colleges or right in his own living room, or traveling to Europe to continue his studies of natural healing techniques. A family man, he regrets that his work too often takes him away from his wife and three children.

For me, my relationship with Dr. D'Adamo has ended an arduous search for a doctor I could trust. Like many people, I was not fully satisfied with the care provided by my family physician. Now, it's gratifying to know that my wife, my baby and I are in the healing hands of someone who has a real understanding of our individual bodies and who can provide us with unerring health care.

Allan Richards

1

I Am a Naturopath

I am a Naturopath and I practice natural healing. What is natural healing? Some believe that it is a way of curing disease with herbal remedies. Others bathe in mineral waters and think that is natural healing. Still others believe natural healing affects the mind and soul, they associate it with practices such as the laying-on-of-hands.

Naturopathy—the natural path of health—is all of these and more. A Naturopath uses many methods of healing, including those that utilize fresh air, the sun, clay, heat, color, sound and food. When people ask me for a quick and simple definition of natural healing, I usually say that it is a way of healing *without the use of drugs*.

Nature's medicine cabinet is filled with safer healing substances than those commonly prescribed by conventional medical practitioners. In fact, many of the powerful drugs and chemicals and harsh, artificial treatments and procedures used in modern medicine can actually be hazardous to your health.

Ironically enough, it was Hippocrates, the ancient Greek physician who is considered the founder of modern medicine, who advised some twenty-five hundred years ago, "Let thy food be thy medicine and thy medicine thy food." Conventional medicine has strayed far from Hippocrates—Naturopaths keep his wisdom alive.

If you were to consult me, I, as a Naturopath, might prescribe various herbs and vitamins. I might recommend that you spend some time in the country, for I agree with Thoreau's faith in Nature's healing powers: "Whenever I need to recreate myself I seek the darkest woods."

However, in this book, I am primarily concerned with the maintenance of your health and well-being through your own *individualized* diet. Food, when used in the right way, can build your body up and keep it strong and vital; when eaten stupidly and indiscriminately, it can weaken your body and help to bring on disease.

In the last decades, there has been an explosion of health-related books. Physical fitness and an abiding American involvement in ecology and conservation have made more and more people question the way they live and the way they eat. "Foodaholics" seek help from such organizations as Weight Watchers and Overeaters Anonymous—and read diet books. There are books on all sorts of weight-loss and health diets: water diets and fasting diets, liquid protein, high protein/low carbohydrate, fruit and vegetable regimens, nucleic acid diets. There are diet books for the commuter, the jogger, the housewife, the business executive, the student and the model.

Aside from the curious regimens the books recommend, they all—even the most popular and acclaimed—have one thing in common: they lose sight of the individual. The conventional diet book does not take into consideration the fact that *you* are different from other individuals reading the book, with a different body and different nutritional needs.

I have held back a long time from writing a book on diet and health simply because I didn't feel that I could provide my readers with the same kind of personal approach I give my patients.

Now, however, I have discovered a way to help you as an individual. I believe that in this book, I can give you what no other diet book or book on Natural Healing has yet provided: a specialized diet plan for your body in your current state of health. Moreover, I will provide you with additional diets to follow after you have begun to experience a renewed sense of health and energy.

Of course, it is a very good idea to seek professional guidance before beginning any diet program. A thorough physical examination and analysis of your current health by your own doctor is a vital first step.

As a Naturopath, I know that a well-nourished body won't easily become susceptible to illness. Nature supplies us with many therapies, but the best treatment for all disease is prevention! Only by selecting those foods that are right for your individual body, will you be able to maintain your strength and health.

Let me tell you about some of the major differences between how the Naturopaths and Allopaths (conventional medical doctors) treat a patient. Allopathic physicians have, for the most part, stopped viewing man as an integral part of his natural environment. They treat disease with expedient synthetic therapies that often do not really get at the cause of an illness. The medical doctor attempts to obliterate invading bacteria or viruses, or to sedate a pain, hoping that the symptoms of the disorder will go away—but I believe that they seldom cure the underlying cause of illness.

Naturopaths know that man has always looked to his environment for foods, herbs, and other natural substances to cure disease and maintain good health. At the dawn of mankind, Neanderthal Man had already begun to use herbs to treat his maladies. In ancient Egypt and in Greco-Roman times, herbs, food and water were used to heal wounds and sickness. In China, five thousand years ago, doctors prescribed foods to prevent disease—and if the patient became sick the doctor had to cure him free of charge!

The Hopi Indians had been practicing Homeopathy, a system of healing that utilizes minute doses of herb and animal substances to produce an effect similar to an illness and thereby neutralize it, hundreds of years before the eighteenth century German physician Dr. Samuel Hahnemann discovered this technique of healing.

A story from Colonial times exemplifies man's ability to find natural cures—long before scientists formalized these remedies. Several years after the settlers arrived in New England, many came down with scurvy: bleeding gums, gray–red blotches on the skin, and profound lassitude. Having marveled at the unusually high level of health enjoyed by their Indian neighbors, they turned to them for medical assistance. The Indians offered the colonists a staple of their diet, wild blueberries and rose hips. Reluctantly, a few of the settlers tried these unfamiliar fruits—and within a few days, they were completely healed. Many years later these natural berries were analyzed and found to be very high in ascorbic acid, Vitamin C, which is both a preventative and cure for scurvy.

Animals have an acute, inborn sense of healing. A sick cat does not eat and curls itself into a ball. This instinctive action stimulates its nervous system, relaying a message to the digestive tract to increase the nutrient supply to the body, thus nourishing and healing the animal.

I am amazed when skeptics scoff at this instinctive ability of the body to heal itself—*vis medicatrix naturae*—once as strong an impulse in man as it remains in animals.

Studies of primitive tribes, such as the Zulu in Africa, reveal that these peoples who live close to Nature were virtually free of the illnesses common among "civilized" man. They ate only such basic foods as grains, fresh fruits and vegetables and small amounts of meat, and drank plenty of water. None of the processed foods with their multitudes of chemical additives found on the dinner table in most American homes were available to these still-primitive communities.

Further studies of tribesmen who had left their villages for the cities and had begun eating commercially processed foods described drastic changes in their health. For the first time, these people succumbed to hardening of the arteries, diabetes and arthritis—the widespread degenerative diseases of civilized man associated with poor diet and health practices.

As a Naturopath, I use many ancient remedies and techniques that come to me from generation upon generation of Natural Healers. I also make use of the modern discoveries made by medical doctors who, disenchanted by conventional drug therapy, have turned to the gentler, more reliable cures of Nature.

My primary method of diagnosis is through the examination of the iris of the eye (see illustrated charts in the Appendix). Iridology, or iris-diagnosis, was first practiced by the Ayurvedic doctors of ancient India and by physicians in China over three thousand years ago. It was brought to a precise science in the last two centuries by European medical doctors who demonstrated that the iris is an exact physiological mirror of the body and the mind.

Iridology can be clearly understood if we realize that every cell, tissue and organ of the body is connected to the brain by the sympathetic nervous system. For example: you touch a flame, the network of nerves relays this action to the brain, pain is registered, and through an automatic reflex—you snatch your hand from the fire. When the brain receives information that any part of the body is altered for any reason—be it trauma, an acidic stomach or an inflamed kidney—it transmits this information via the nervous system to the iris. The myriad nerve filaments spread all around the iris correspond to particular tissues or organs within the body.

Heart damage for instance, would be recorded as either a minute white line denoting a recent or acute attack or a gray ovule indicating a chronic problem at approximately three o'clock (visualize the iris as a clock face) in the right eye. An infected liver would appear as either a white line or gray ovule (depending upon the severity of the condition) at about 7:45 in the left eye, and a malfunctioning ovary would show up at about 5:25 in the left eye.

These are only examples of the findings revealed by iridology and I beg you, don't try self-diagnosis! If you cannot resist examining your own irises and discover lines or ovules, don't panic and assume that disease is present. It takes many years of experience in examining thousands of patients to learn how to read and interpret the signs of the eye correctly.

Since I possess this experience, a thorough diagnosis of the eyes tells me if any organs are stressed, what the body's level of toxicity is, and what illnesses the patient has suffered in the past. I have found that even if these illnesses were treated by drugs, the signs still appear in the eyes because drugs only alleviate symptoms and do not heal the underlying cause of the disorder.

Most important, this diagnostic technique shows me which parts of the patient's body are nutritionally deficient and then I know which foods and herbs will rebuild the body into health.

In addition to recommending specialized diets, vitamins and herbal therapy, I also make use of other time-proven remedies. Where applicable, I use a variety of herbal baths and clay therapy because water and clay draw toxic wastes from the body, hastening the regeneration of tissue and organs. I use homeopathic remedies to help stimulate an organ and rebalance its natural processes. To relieve muscular pain, I may use acupuncture, massage or bone manipulation. Color Therapy (see Chapter 11) is beneficial to a devitalized organ or tissue and can precipitate psychological changes. I often prescribe one or more of the twelve tissue salts in order either to maintain proper condition or to cure the various ailments that result from an imbalance in these vital constituents of the human body.

However, the cornerstone of my method of healing is the individualized diet—and I will teach you how to find the nutrition that will bring you health, energy and well-being.

Unlike many conventional medical practitioners, I do not treat symptoms of disease—I hunt out the underlying causes of the disorder that are creating the variety of reactions and symptoms. I treat the whole patient, body and mind inextricably interwoven, applying what is commonly called the holistic principle.

My files are filled with hundreds of case histories of patients who had come to me suffering symptoms of illnesses that had never been properly diagnosed or cured because they had never been examined or treated holistically and naturally.

Let me tell you about one such case, a young man who had been experiencing depressions, migraine headaches with accompanying nausea, low vitality and a tendency toward alcoholism. His medical doctor, who had not diagnosed the underlying cause of these disorders, had provided him with a palliative to ease each symptom: an antidepressant for his despondency, codeine and aspirin for his headaches, antacids for his nausea. The drugs brought him relief—until their effects wore off.

When I examined this young man's eyes, I saw signs that his pancreas was severely stressed and under constant demand to secrete insulin. I could then diagnose that he suffered from hypoglycemia (low blood sugar).

I created a special diet for this young man, one that put much less strain on his pancreas by vastly reducing his carbohydrate intake, eliminating such foods as sugar, honey, and many grains and cereals. To help repair damaged tissue and regenerate his physical vitality, I increased his protein consumption, adding a serving of animal protein (chicken, fish or veal) as well as soybean curd (tofu) three times a day.

After eight months on the high-protein/low-carbohydrate diet, the patient's depressions, headaches and nausea ceased. He regained a tremendous amount of energy, and though he still drank beer occasionally, his body no longer craved the carbohydrates in alcohol and his drinking was no longer a problem.

Dr. Hahnemann, the founder of Homeopathy, wrote in his book, *Organon of Medicine:*

The human body is, in its living state, a unity, a complete and rounded whole. Every sensation, every manifestation of force, every interrelation of the material of one part is intimately concerned with the sensation, force, manifestation and interrelations of all the other parts; no part suffers without involving all the rest in suffering and alteration.

Put more simply, the whole body and each of its parts work in conjunction and have a direct effect upon one another.

Now, I will take the advice of George Bernard Shaw who wrote that "principles without programs are platitudes" and show you, as I have so many of my patients, how to find the diet that is right for *you*.

2

The Way to Health

Many people think of health as the pot of gold at the end of the rainbow and consider illness to be inevitable. Nothing could be further from the truth. It actually takes more effort and hard work to make yourself sick than it does to stay healthy! Medical doctors are astounded: they consider this simplistic. I know that my formulations are not conventional thinking—but very little natural healing *is* conventional. As a practicing Naturopath, I work closely with Nature and have a special understanding of her ways.

Let me repeat: Illness requires time and the exertion of great energy on your part. Illness is the quirk of Nature. Good health, however, can be readily attained and be everyone's good fortune.

The ways to health and the causes of illness are controversial even among medical doctors, and have probably always been so since man first sought healing. Naturopaths and Allopaths understand health and illness in different ways and therefore have different approaches to healing. Most Allopaths believe germs and viruses *cause* infectious disease. Naturopaths see the presence of germs in infectious and degenerative illnesses as a *result* of a weakened body condition brought on by poor nutrition or mental or emotional stress. In the Naturopathic view, germs are the effect of disease, not the cause.

Many medical doctors also cite such factors as heredity, immunology and environmental pollution in their explanations of the causes of disease. I agree that all these can be contributing factors, but they are not usually the main causes. Look at the statistics on the rise of major diseases in this country. Over 40 percent of all deaths are attributed to heart disease; fifty million Americans suffer with arthritis; forty-five million have some sort of respiratory disease such as asthma, bronchitis or emphysema. Doesn't this indicate that conventional medicine has a poor track record in interpreting, preventing and curing major illnesses?

If I were a potential patient of a medical doctor, the following quote in the *New York Times,* April 17, 1979, would certainly affect my faith and confidence in my physician. Dr. William Barclay, who is editor of the prestigious *Journal of the American Medical Association,* wrote that:

The fact that a [medical] doctor using the word "cure" does not mean it in the strict sense of total removal, without any chance of recurring, should not be taken pessimistically. The concept of disease control is just as satisfactory as cure from the patient's standpoint. He has a reasonable chance of living a normal life free of symptoms of that disease.

Speaking for myself, I would want to know that my sickness was completely removed from my body and not just "under control." Many of my patients have come to me because they, too, wanted a *total cure.* In true healing, there is no such thing as a "reasonable chance" of living a normal life: a person is either healed and healthy—or not. This can only be accomplished by cleansing and nourishing the body, regenerating it to full strength so that it is no longer prone to illness.

To understand the causes of diseases, it would be helpful if we considered precisely how the body, as a biological organism, works. In the sixteenth century, the Swiss physician Paracelsus observed that "the body is a conglomeration of chemical matter." Three centuries later, the great German pathologist Rudolf Virchow argued that the health of the body is dependent upon the health of its cells, and that the chemical makeup of each cell is directly affected by the food it ingests. Virchow was the first scientist to emphasize that the cell is the basic unit of the body and his work has inspired countless medical doctors and bacteriologists. Later investigators determined that the ability of nerve, muscle and sensory cells (such as those in the eyes and nose) to function normally depended upon their having a proper balance of minerals, protein compounds and vitamins.

Cells have two main activities in the body: internal functions such as digestion, circulation of nutrients, respiration and reproduction, which are necessary for their survival, and external duties as part of a larger system of the body, such as tissue, muscle, or an organ.

If we view a cell as a microcosmic part of the entire body, one can easily see that a cell must be fed certain substances from its environment, such as oxygen, protein particles and glucose. Similarly, the cell must eliminate waste products, such as carbon dioxide and uric acid. The interchange of nutrients and air is negotiated by intercellular fluids, which can be thought of as waterways through which boats deliver goods, take on cargo, and sail out back to sea.

If the chemistry of these fluids is polluted with any extraneous wastes, such as an inordinate amount of uric acid crystals or with mucus, the transference of food and oxygen will be obstructed. The effects of the following salts on a cell membrane suggest how easily cellular functions can be disturbed. Calcium chloride thickens the cell membrane and blocks the passage of food into the cell. Sodium chloride (table salt), on the other hand, softens this thin cell membrane and interferes with the cell's ability to absorb the proper substances. The effects of salts upon cell composition was demonstrated more than eighty years ago when it was proved that any deficiency of inorganic minerals not only drastically alters the health of cells in the body but of the units the cells comprise, such as tissues, muscles, organs or entire bodily systems.

Before the nineteenth-century scientists Pasteur and Koch formulated the germ theory of disease, the investigator Bechamp accepted Virchow's findings that disease begins when there is any alteration in the normal chemical state of the cell and its environment. Bechamp explained this formulation by pointing out that a weakened cell has less resistance and natural immunity, and thus attracts bacteria. "Disease," he insisted, "is produced by germs seeking their natural habitat—diseased tissue—and not by spontaneous germ action."

But what is it exactly that lowers the body's resistance and creates this "diseased habitat?" If we think of the human body as a sublime machine of Nature, we can understand that it requires fuel in order to run and that the quality of the fuel affects its performance.

As I have said, cells require minerals, vitamins, proteins and various other compounds and these substances are obtainable from fruits, vegetables, grains and meat. However, each person is different, with subtly different chemistry, varying rates of metabolism and hormonal balance and not all foods have the same effect upon all individuals. For example, dairy products (eggs, cheese, milk) are mucus-forming in many people. The protein in cheese and milk, casein, is not easily assimilated by these people. It irritates the delicate mucous membrane that line the digestive tract, causing it to secrete a white substance known as mucus. I have discovered that once the mucus is released, it can circulate throughout your body and envelop and clog cells in any organ. When this occurs in the lungs, for example, the lung cells begin to "choke" and can no longer function normally because they are weakened. A weakened organ has a lower level of resistance and is therefore prone to infection, in this case, to such respiratory diseases as bronchitis or pneumonia.

Other food has different effects on the body. Too much red meat in your diet can increase the uric acid in your blood. Uric acid, which can be poison, is normally filtered from the body by the kidneys. An excessive amount of uric acid can overwhelm the kidney cells, clogging and choking them and reducing their filtration ability. Once weakened, I believe that the kidneys, like the lungs, can be invaded by bacteria and an ailment such as nephritis can result.

Ordinary medical science does not generally attribute these types of disorders to the food you eat. A respiratory infection is not linked to the accumulation of mucus from the overconsumption of dairy products and uric acid from red meats is not cited as the cause of kidney impairment. Your consumption of nutritionless processed foods such as white flour, refined sugar or TV dinners, all of which retard enzymatic action in your stomach and cause retention of toxic wastes, is not recognized as the cause of many of your illnesses. But in spite of conventional medical indifference to these things, it is a fact that toxins from these foods alter your cellular environment, just as the accumulation of mucus or uric acid does, lowering your resistance and weakening your tissues.

For many years you have eaten inferior foods and foods that your body cannot properly assimilate and this has made your body weak and prone to infectious and degenerative disease.

Basically, there are two kinds of diseases, acute and chronic. I believe that an acute disease is usually brought on by your body's violent efforts to throw off wastes that have not been properly eliminated and which are upsetting normal cellular function. An acute disease can be thought of as an effort of the body to cleanse itself.

If your body is not assisted in ridding itself of these toxins through diet or certain detoxifying treatments, your problem, in my experience, can develop into a chronic condition. In other words, if the accumulation of mucus in your chest which is now causing a wheezing cough is not discharged from your body, it could eventually result in a chronic case of asthma. I have found that a chronic disease is caused by an accumulation of waste matter over the years.

You may not always be so fortunate as to have an acute disease acting as an alarm and warning you that something is wrong in your body. A chronic disease, such as arthritis or arteriosclerosis, can often develop quietly without any telltale signs. Though you may have thought of yourself as the picture of health, one day you may find, much to your surprise, that you have an unexpected and serious illness.

Whether you have an acute or chronic disease, your medical doctor will probably treat you with drugs. An antibiotic would probably be prescribed for a bacterial chest condition, such as pneumonia, or for a kidney infection like nephritis. Without recognizing that the mucus in your lungs or the uric acid in your kidneys is causing your disorder, the Allopath's *modus operandi* would be to vanquish the bacteria and drive the infection from your body. While the bacteria may be dealt a deadly blow, the true underlying cause of your illness, which I believe to be the weakened body environment that has not been regenerated, has been overlooked. In my experience, most patients treated in this fashion are likely to experience a recurrence of the same or of a related ailment.

Let me tell you about one of my patients, a fashion photographer who had severe arthritic pains in his neck and shoulders. After only weeks on the dairy-free diet that I created for him, he could turn his neck without the customary gnawing aches and rest his head comfortably on his pillow at night for the first time in two years! Suddenly, he was a changed person. Instead of walking hunched over with a scowl on his face, he now held his body erect and had an attractive, cheerful expression.

Believing that he was healed, he went off his diet and back to his old eating habits, including his daily lunch of a prosciutto and cheese sandwich. Within days, his aches and pains returned. A "specialist" put him in traction for a week, gave him cortisone shots and prescribed codeine to kill the pain. Like the young man with hypoglycemia I told you about, the photographer was relieved of his discomforts—until the drugs wore off.

I repeat: drugs relieve only symptoms, and they do so at great cost. When an antibiotic such as penicillin is administered to your

22

body, it eliminates invading bacteria by weakening the cell walls of multiplying bacteria. Deprived of these rigid walls, the bacteria die. However, in addition to destroying invading bacteria, an antibiotic can eliminate strains of bacteria that normally dwell in your body. When these bacteria are kept in check through competition with other strains, their numbers are relatively small and they are harmless. However, when bacteria are destroyed indiscriminately by an antibiotic, only a few strains may survive and they can reproduce wildly. This kind of reaction, called a suprainfection, can cause severe infection which may even result in death.

It has been estimated that over half of all illnesses suffered in America today are caused by the use of drugs. A seemingly innocent drug that you may use for symptomatic relief can unleash a vicious chain reaction of disharmony and disorder in your body. For instance, you may take some common over-the-counter antihistamine for a cold. On the side of the package there is a warning of possible harmful side effects. You take this and within a few days your cold may be contained. However, during the "cure," an organ, such as a lung, may become irritated. You go to your doctor, who diagnoses your condition and prescribes another drug for your chest problem. The great majority of prescription drugs carry no warning of any potential danger, although they too can cause adverse side effects. Literature on the possible side effects of a drug prescribed by a medical doctor can only be obtained if you request this information from your pharmacist!

Your lung tissue may soon be healed by the prescribed medication, but that drug may have caused another organ to become irritated. Another drug is then prescribed and taken, and then another and another, perpetuating the chain of illnesses. Finally, when drug therapy fails, the only solution may be the surgical removal of a diseased part of your body.

In their book, *The Swine Flu Affair,* Harvard professors Richard E. Neustadt and Harvey V. Fineberg indict this vaccination program for being a hasty effort that caused many drug-related disorders. The authors charge that the side effects incurred nationwide—including some deaths—could have been reduced if Dr. Spencer, then head of the Center for Disease Control, and Dr. Cooper, then Assistant Secretary of Health, had not pushed the vaccination program through without weighing its potential dangers.

As I have told you before, Naturopaths heal by the proper use of substances basic to man: his food. By eliminating impure and unhealthful foods such as refined sugar and white flour and ingesting a simple regimen of fresh fruits and vegetables, whole grains and, where appropriate, meats, the body is helped to purify itself and to rebuild its weakened parts. I have yet to see a person who had changed his diet to these more nutritious foods fail to recover a good deal of his health. Furthermore, because a Naturopath truly understands the nutritional values of food, he recommends only those which have a healing effect on the different organs, tissues and bones.

For example, he may suggest that a person with a kidney inflammation or kidney stones eat dandelion leaves or drink dandelion tea to help eliminate clogged wastes and excess uric acid. To someone with arthritis, he may recommend raw celery stalks to dissolve the inorganic calcium deposits in his body. He may suggest chamomile tea to relax the abdominal muscles of a person suffering stomach cramps, okra to help improve digestion and the elimination of bodily wastes, or pumpkin seeds to strengthen a weakened or inflamed prostate gland.

The relationship of foods to different parts of the body can be more clearly understood if we take a look at man's position in the food chain. The Bible says that God made man from dust, and man is literally, as well as metaphorically, composed of the elements and minerals found within the earth. Moreover, a constant and complete supply of these minerals is fundamental to health.

Obviously, we cannot make direct use of these mineral substances existing in the earth because our bodies are not equipped to convert them into assimilable compounds. But, plants are capable of just that! A plant absorbs nutrients from the soil and when we eat these plants, be they vegetable, fruit or grain, we receive these minerals in a form that our bodies *can* digest and use.

A wider variety of nutrients is obtained when we eat meats from such animals as chicken, lamb, or fish, which have been nurtured through eating plants. Here we receive both the minerals absorbed by the plants plus the complete amino-acid proteins which are formed in animals.

Each plant or animal that we eat provides us with different nutritive substances. For example, tomatoes and carrots are rich in silicon, which is essential for the health of connective tissues such as ligaments and muscles. Citrus fruits and watercress are good sources of potassium, which is vital for proper kidney function. Fish, cabbage, and dried beans provide sulphur, which invigorates the bloodstream and is necessary to the healthy functioning of your nervous system.

Any deficiency of the basic minerals will weaken your body, lower your natural resistance and increase your susceptibility to disease. However, I have found that illness can be cured and health and vitality restored and maintained when the proper nutrients are supplied to your body. This does not mean adhering to some bizarre diet or starving yourself to lose a few pounds by denying yourself the pleasures of eating. All it means is eating those foods that are compatible with *your* body.

Nature's power to regenerate Herself can be illustrated by the story of Jamaica Bay, which surrounds New York's busy Kennedy Airport. Dr. René Dubos, the Nobel Prize-winning microbiologist, has written of this area, which was once so contaminated and barren that no birds or fish had thrived there for over fifty years. Recently, however, a New York Parks Commissioner began to plant trees there, pines and bayberries. As the trees grew, birds began to return—then fish—and soon rabbits and squirrels were inhabiting this estuary. As Nature is resilient, so is the human body, which struggles to throw off toxins and heal itself.

Even though most people who come to see me are in a state of ill health with their systems out of balance and their blood and joints laden with toxic deposits, I have found that after a short period on a specialized diet they begin to experience a renewed feeling of health.

A young married woman came to me after she had consulted several gynecologists about an abnormality in her reproductive organs. All these doctors had given her the same diagnosis: diseased fallopian tubes. Their recommendations had been for a hysterectomy, an operation which would remove her entire reproductive system. In despair at the thought of not being able to have children, as a last resort she decided to give natural healing a try.

When I examined her, I found her body to be highly acidic and stressed, so I created a high-protein soy diet for her. I eliminated citrus fruits and wheat products and limited her consumption of meat, because the high acid content of these foods would continue to have a debilitating effect on her tissues. The more alkaline soy products would not be corrosive and the high protein would help to rebuild her malfunctioning organs. In addition to this specialized diet, I prescribed a series of colonic irrigations for this patient. Within four months she was completely healed, and the joy of motherhood, which had almost been stolen from her, became a reality a year-and-a-half later when she gave birth to a son.

Let me tell you about one more case. A mother brought her daughter to me suffering with an acute inflammation of the appendix. The recommendation of the general practitioner they had previously consulted had been immediate removal of the appendix to prevent internal poisoning. The appendix was swollen and caused sharp sticking pains in the girl's lower groin.

After examination, I did not believe that her condition was serious enough to warrant the unnecessary risks and trauma of surgery. I immediately put the girl on a strict vegetarian diet and required her to drink twelve glasses of water daily. In addition, she underwent colon therapy to cleanse the ascending portion of this organ, which was clogged with wastes that pressed down upon the appendix and irritated it. I gave the patient a small box with an infrared light mounted within it and recommend that she hold it over the painful area for fifteen minutes a day. Within a week, the pains ceased, the swelling abated, and the patient's appendix returned to its normal size and shape. (A reader using this technique should be careful to avoid overheating the box, which might cause scorching or fire.)

Healing is really a simple art, primarily a matter of providing the body with the specific nourishment that it needs to sustain its natural strength and vitality. Of course, the Natural cure is not an instant remedy, for Nature takes time in rebuilding health and returning the body to well-being. But this I do promise you, the Natural cure is gentle, long-lasting and respectful of your entire body.

3

The D'Adamo Discovery

Many years ago, when I first practiced Natural Healing, I began to question the routine Naturopathic techniques in which I had been trained. A Naturopath, like a medical doctor or any professional, can arrive at the point where he takes what he has learned, adapts it, and carries it further. I must confess that I have always been a maverick, and although I learned and accepted what I had been taught, I continued to question and look for other ways—sometimes unheard-of ways—of healing.

Generally speaking, most Naturopathic practitioners recognize that each man and woman is a unique creation with a special assortment of cells, tissues, nerves, hereditary traits and a unique psychological temperament. Nevertheless, these practitioners believed that the same foods were suited to all patients and that these patients could be treated for the same illnesses in the same ways!

The majority of Naturopaths considered man to be herbivorous and believed that a vegetarian regimen was his correct nutritional path in health and in illness. Other healers believed that daily allowances of the Basic Four (meat, dairy, vegetables and fruits) provided the perfectly balanced diet. Although these practitioners disagreed about diets, they were in perfect agreement that all humanity could be treated as one.

Unlike my colleagues, I believed that no two people on the face of the earth were alike; no two people have the same fingerprints, lip-prints or voices, and even identical twins do not share all physical characteristics. Because I felt that all people were different from one another, I thought that it was ridiculous that all people should eat the same foods. Why should individuals be expected to be able to tolerate or derive similar nutritional value from the same kind of foods, and how could they be healed in the exact same way? It became clear to me that since each person was housed in a special body with different strengths, weaknesses, sensitivities and nutritional requirements, the only way to maintain health or cure illness was to accommodate a patient's diet to his specific individual needs.

This thinking brought me into conflict with the therapeutic practices of my fellow Naturopaths. It defied the traditional methods of healing I had been taught at some of the most prominent institutes and clinics in Europe. Despite the differences in nutritional programs, all patients in these clinics were treated with standardized diets and therapies with no consideration of the inherent physical uniqueness of each individual.

At the Kneipp Institute, where I received my basic training in Natural Healing, arthritis was treated with a strict vegetarian diet and no patient was allowed beef, pork, chicken, fish, or dairy products. Arthritis was believed to be caused by the inability of the kidneys to flush toxic wastes and mucus from the body so that these substances were reabsorbed by the blood, which circulated and deposited them into various tissues and caused swelling, aches and pains. Therefore, all meals consisted of vegetable salads and fruit cups, which would remove impurities from the bloodstream, help purify the kidneys and make the filtration of wastes from the body again possible. When the cleansing action of the fruits and vegetables reduced toxicity, swelling and pain would abate.

Yet, during these treatments I often observed that not all

patients had the same response. The diet suited some well, and these patients maintained a bright disposition as their condition improved. Others, however, were less capable of sustaining their strength on such a regimen. They became pale, weak and lifeless and showed such side effects as fatigue, mental depression and muscular atrophy. Some patients would describe themselves as feeling "disconnected," and a small percentage of those treated would be entirely unresponsive.

I saw similar effects at other institutes where treatment was uniformly administered. At one clinic in Switzerland, where I later studied and practiced, the standard treatment for arthritis was a vegetarian diet augmented by dairy producs such as cheese, yogurt, milk and butter. Here again, different patients had different responses to treatment. Some remained strong and alert while healing, but others suffered from sluggishness, despondency and disconnectedness. Some patients did not get better, and some actually got worse.

These disparate patient reactions were not limited to arthritis. Whenever an illness—arteriosclerosis, low blood sugar, or gout—was treated with a standardized diet, similar results occurred. Even though the cure rate was often as high as 80 percent, and the methods were superior to drug therapy, I felt that a true treatment should heal all people, not just some.

When I returned to the United States to set up my practice, I knew that I would have to break away from many of the traditional methods of Natural Healing in order to find a way to cure more than 80 percent of my patients. I believed that I could cure 100 percent, if I could discover a way to treat each person as an individual, providing a diet and treatment perfectly suited to each patient.

This may strike you as very egotistical, but healing *is* a God-given gift, something you have a feeling for and have always known that you possess. As a boy, I was always trying to heal sick dogs and cats, injured trees and dying plants, while others my age were out playing ball. Although admittedly it took me years to understand why my interests were so different from those of my peers, I kept using my ability to heal animals, graft broken branches back onto trees and make weak plants flourish.

I do believe healing ability comes from within, and the more closely I listened to and followed my intuition, the better I was able to heal my pets and plants. Throughout my career, these feelings have guided me, "telling" me which foods and treatments were required by my patients.

As a young physician, I had a strong feeling that somewhere within the body there must be an organic signpost, a biological feature that could differentiate one person's nutritional needs from those of another. Of course, I wasn't the first doctor to try to explain the differences between human beings. Throughout history, many attempts have been made by scientists and religious men as well as by doctors, to classify people by distinguishing physical characteristics.

For example, Hippocrates taught that four body humors, blood, yellow bile, black bile and phlegm determined man's state of health. He believed that man's temperament was determined by the predominant humor: sanguine (blood), choleric (yellow bile), melancholic (black bile) and phlegmatic (phlegm). In ancient India, the Ayurvedic doctors categorized patients into three types of "faults," each of which represented an aspect of bodily imbalance. The psychiatrist Carl Jung believed that people tended to either introversion or extroversion. Both Catholics and Hindus divide humanity into two great groups: those who find enlightenment or salvation through action and those who follow the contemplative way.

One of the most comprehensive systems of classification was devised by Dr. William Sheldon. In his exhaustive work, *Atlas of Men,* he corelated body types with psychological and spiritual factors. According to Dr. Sheldon, the endomorph, who is round and fat, is characterized by a fear of being alone, an indiscriminate friendliness and a passion for food. The mesomorph, who is big-boned and brawny, is competitive, loves physical power and is indifferent to the pain and the sensitivities of others. The ectomorph, a small-boned and frail person, is overly sensitive, shy and nervous, and is often highly creative and/or devoutly religious.

However none of these systems of classification corelates an individual's physical, psychological and spiritual habits with his dietary needs. True, both the Bible and the Hindu Book of Wisdom, the Bhagavad-Gītā, relate food to physical and spiritual health, but never specifically with individual differences in mind.

I intended to gain insight into the way different bodies utilized nutrients both in nourishing and in healing themselves. Was there a signpost to guide me? If so, what?

During my training years in Germany, I had heard of several doctors who had been trying to relate the kinds of food a person should eat to his blood type. I understood that these investigations developed out of experiments by German doctors who, during the war, had tried to devise specialized diets for soldiers that would provide maximum nutrition for a minimum of food.

The discovery that not all people had the same type of blood was made in 1900 by Dr. Karl Landsteiner, the great Austrian pathologist who later became a U.S. citizen. In 1930, he received the Nobel Prize for his work. Roughly speaking, what Dr. Landsteiner demonstrated was that red blood cells (erythrocytes) in some individuals produced a substance called an antibody when mixed with the red blood cells taken from other individuals. Landsteiner then proved that humans could be classified into four groups on the basis of these naturally occurring antibodies to the red blood cells of individuals in other groups. For example, serum from group-A individuals caused the cells of group-B individuals to form clumps while serum from group-B subjects caused the cells of group-A subjects to mass and clump together (agglutinate). In contrast, serum from group-O subjects caused both A and B cells to mass while neither A nor B sera could agglutinate O cells.

The fourth group, AB, was found soon after the discovery of groups A, B and O. This group, which represents about 5 percent of the population, possesses cells which are massed or clumped by sera from group A, B and O individuals but do not agglutinate the cells of any of the other groups.

This all sounds—and is—complex, but the implications are far-reaching. The discovery of these four distinct blood types saved countless lives because, now that blood could be matched, transfusions became a valuable part of medical treatment. It is now known that to receive the benefits of blood transfusion in the treatment of blood loss owing to surgery or trauma or other conditions, the blood given must be of the same type as that of the patient. If blood from a type-A individual is, for example, given to a patient with type-B blood, serious, even fatal consequences will result.

I was fully aware of the importance of blood typing, and indeed the actual procedure of determining an individual's group had become a routine matter. However, it was during this often-practiced laboratory procedure that my inspiration occurred. Blood, I knew, controls body temperature, determines immunity against disease, circulates oxygen, eliminates gaseous wastes and carries nutrients to all parts of the body. Perhaps, I thought, blood also determines the types of nutrients the body was capable of assimilating. In an intuitive leap, or a lucky guess, I hypothesized that a person's blood type, A, B, O or AB determined his nutritional needs.

Almost all scientific investigation, after all, begins with a hypothesis, a profound belief that one has discovered a truth of nature. After the original hypothesis comes years of careful research and investigation designed to prove or disprove the original assumption.

And so, many years ago I began my investigation of the nature of different blood types and their relationship to diet. I studied the response of people with type-A blood to a vegetarian regimen, and how type-O people reacted to a diet consisting of the Basic Four. Carefully, I scrutinized reactions to such potentially mucus-forming foods as dairy products and to foods made from wheat, which are potentially acid-forming.

For example, when I saw a reaction, such as an increase in abdominal acidity or a sensitizing of the skin, I reduced or eliminated all acid-forming foods from the diet. When such effects as lethargy and midday fatigue developed, I increased the allowance of animal proteins and dairy products. I studied my patients continually, watching for specific reactions to food and for reactions common to people of the same blood type.

Each patient was essentially a blind study that could support or disprove my assumption, because all patients of one blood type had to share a common pattern to validate my hypothesis. If patients with the same blood type reacted to the same foods in the same way, I had my signpost. If the patients did not react in this fashion, I had but an interesting theory.

Results came quickly. In the first one hundred patients studied, I noted a definite trend. People with type-A blood manufactured mucus and catarrh when digesting dairy products and animal products. My studies showed that these people maintained their best level of health on a vegetarian diet, and in fact, were the only blood type capable of deriving all their nutritional requirements from a totally vegetarian regimen.

I discovered that people with type-O blood reacted to food in an opposite fashion to those with type A. Type-O people had a more dynamic and vigorous body and were not able to derive their protein needs from a vegetarian diet. These people required daily allowances of meat and dairy products—which did not form mucus in their bodies—to meet their physical needs.

I continued diagnosing patients, gathering information, and recording the tendencies of the different blood types. My investigation of five hundred patients continued to support my theory. However, occasionally I would have a patient who did not fit into the pattern. I was confused and thrown off course. Was this a deviation from a blood type, or had I failed to observe something vital about the patient? I discovered the answer after putting these patients on a generalized diet and correcting some of their illnesses. After this had been done, the patient's body would then respond according to the pattern I had observed in others of his blood type. The disorder had "perverted" the patient's body.

For example, a type B, whose body had been sensitive to wheat products, and who had been producing large amounts of mucus from dairy products—reacting like a type A—was later able to digest and assimilate these foods after his blood had been purified of circulating mucus and his kidneys strengthened so that they could filter wastes from his body.

As I continued to study, my signpost became less of a theory and more of a reality. I tested thousands of patients and developed a broader understanding of each blood type; its nutritional requirements, physical characteristics and psychological makeup. After twenty years of diagnosing, examining, and working with patients, I believe that I have successfully demonstrated that my hypothesis, once an intuitive feeling, is a truth of Nature that applies to all people.

The consistency of my results led me to understand why there had been such a disparity in the reactions of patients to the standardized diets in the health clinics. The strict vegetarian diet administered by those at the Kneipp Institute to heal arthritis was the appropriate treatment for patients with type-A blood, because these people could sustain themselves on such a regimen. However, people with type-O blood suffered fatigue and loss of strength, because they did not receive the supply of animal protein necessary to their well-being.

The vegetarian/dairy diet prescribed for arthritis at a famous clinic in Switzerland affected people with type-O blood in the same way because it, also, did not provide the animal protein they required. Moreover, patients with type-A blood, who were already catarrhal, incurred an increase in mucus when they ate cheese, yogurt, milk and butter, thus worsening their condition.

A further discovery that grew from my many years of studying the relationship of blood types to nutritional needs was that certain physiological conditions are associated with each type. For example, most people with type-O blood have a strong muscular body and are very active physically. On the other hand, my studies have shown that types A and AB are exactly opposite to type-O people, with trimmer physiques and less dynamic, more passive bodies. People with type-B blood tend to have medium builds, neither so brawny as the O, nor so trim as the A and AB.

People have different physical energy-vitality levels, and this, too, I have found can be directly corelated with their blood types. I developed and use the expression "vibrational body" to describe and categorize the energy-vitality level. (This should not be confused with the actual vibrational level of the body, which is a measure of its electromagnetic energy.)

I have found that the different blood groups naturally fall into one of the three energy-level types: highly charged and active, moderately active, or passive. People with type-O blood usually have a high vibrational body, that is, an inherently energetic and active one. Types A and AB are usually passive in their energy-vitality level and therefore can be described as having low-vibrational bodies. People with type-B blood fall between the two extremes in their energy-vitality level (just as they do in their physical makeup) and can be described as having medial vibrational bodies.

I have rated foods by their vibrational level in accordance to the type of blood group and vibrational body with which they correspond. For example, dairy products and animal proteins are high vibrational foods because they are foods that people with a high vibrational body (type O) can readily assimilate without forming large quantities of mucus or acidity.

Vegetables, fruits and grains are best suited for those with A and AB blood who have low-vibrational bodies, therefore, I have named them low-vibrational foods.

This does not mean that a person with type-O blood with a high vibrational body should not eat low-vibrational foods such as vegetables or fruits. He may eat low-vibrational foods in addition to the large quantities of high-vibrational animal proteins, which are necessary to maintain his well-being. In contrast, an A or AB blood type, who is passive and not able to readily digest animal proteins, should, in most instances, eat only fruits, vegetables and grains: the low-vibrational foods.

Therefore, in determining a patient's diet, I prescribe only those foods which are in harmony with his blood type and his vibrational body. Foods which are not in harmony with the body's vibration do not supply the required nutrients and cannot be assimilated, therefore they will weaken and stress the patient's organs, produce toxicity, and in my experience, cause a degenerative disease.

Generally speaking, of course, there are foods which should be avoided by *everyone* regardless of their blood type. Foods made of refined flours or those containing sugar or chemical additives (white bread, sweets, pastries, jams, soda, canned foods and frozen dinners) can cause a broad range of disorders from tooth decay to, perhaps, cancer. Beef and pork products, which have a high purine content, aid in the formation of uric acid which can contribute to muscular and joint pain.

I have found that even such vegetables as spinach and beets should be eaten sparingly by everyone. It is my experience that too much spinach can lead to a calcium deficiency that can cause aches and swelling of the joints, gum diseases and brittle bones. I also believe that old beets, which have an exceedingly high starch content, can significantly raise blood-sugar levels, thus aggravating or contributing to hypoglycemia.

Even when you eat foods that are wholesome and potentially beneficial, such as grains, various fruits and vegetables, soy products and seeds such as pumpkin or sunflower—you must always consider how these foods will be used in *your* body.

Many people believe that since God gave us such a wide variety of foods, they must all be good for us! However, one man's food may be another man's poison, and only by knowing which foods are best suited for your body can you attain health and well-being.

4

The D'Adamo Diets

You probably already know what your blood type is. It will be a part of your medical records, which are kept by any practitioners you have consulted. However, if you do not remember whether you are an A, B, AB or O, you can easily get this vital information by either requesting it from your medical records or by having your blood typed by a health practitioner, a clinic, or a blood-doner program (such as that run by the Red Cross). The process is painless, quick, and either inexpensive or free. Obviously, if you are to benefit from these diets, you must be sure of your blood type!

As I have told you before, I prescribe special kinds of diets, different from the basic ones for the well person, to those patients who are suffering an illness and those who, while not sick, still are not enjoying their natural high energy level and sense of perfect well-being. In this chapter, however, I would like to describe the physical and psychological characteristics of the different blood types and suggest the proper diet that will enable each group to achieve maximum well-being. These are diets for people currently in a reasonably balanced state of health.

TYPE A

A person with type-A blood, let's call him or her the "A," has a highly sensitive body and is usually naturally intelligent with an active and probing mind. He has strong reasoning power, and can solve complex problems. Because of his acute sensitivity, his creative potential is also very high.

As I have mentioned, the A has a low-vibrational body and tends to be physically inactive. (By low-vibrational, I don't mean to imply good or bad; it is a neutral word. Perhaps "harmonics" best describes what I mean by vibrational.) Many A's, however, my studies have shown, have an overstimulated thyroid gland which heightens their metabolic rate and tends to make them think and perform as physically active persons. When this occurs, the A is being stimulated by nervous kinetic energy, instead of a calmer, more centered physical vitality. This produces a tremendous amount of tension and these A's are impatient, restless, and unable to achieve deep sleep, often moving about a great deal throughout the night. Many walk or talk in their sleep. These A's very probably have never experienced their true natural energy.

Because the A has a low-vibrational body, his nutritional path should be vegetarianism: fruits, grains and vegetables. Animal products, such as beef, pork, veal, chicken, and fish and dairy products, such as cheese, milk, yogurt and eggs, are highly mucus-forming within his body, and should be avoided. Whole-wheat products, which are acid-forming in the A, should be eaten sparingly, once or twice a week, or, preferably, not at all. Grains and breads made of the alkaline-forming soy products are more beneficial to his body, because they are readily digested and do not have a corrosive effect on his body's organs. When selecting vegetables and fruits, the A should choose those that tend to be more alkaline-forming to prevent an increase of acidity in his body.

Some vegetables the A's may want in their diet include leafy greens such as: lettuce, beet greens, collards, Swiss chard and kale; watercress, asparagus, broccoli, carrots (boiled or steamed),

40

fennel, okra, cucumbers, celery, squash, beans and potatoes. Tomatoes, which are too acidic for the A, should be avoided or eaten only occasionally, no more than once a week. Avocados, which are rich in oil, should be eaten sparingly. He should avoid red and white cabbage, which can cause excessive flatulence, and lentils, which are difficult to digest and too highly concentrated in iron for his body.

His fruit selection may include: papaya, strawberries, blueberries, grapefruits, cantaloupe, peaches, apricots, dark Italian plums, Bing cherries and watermelon. Oranges, tangerines and apples should be avoided (or limited to one a week) because they are too acidic. If he believes he must have orange or apple juice it should be diluted with water.

In switching over to a vegetarian diet, the A should proceed *slowly* and *gradually*. A sudden change of diet, any diet, can shock the body or cause undue mental stress. Some people are professional enthusiasts, and jump into a new diet with sheer and utter abandon; but like those people who try to kick a smoking or drinking habit overnight, they soon enough return to their old ways. Therefore change should be slow. The A may take six months to a year to work into a new regimen if necessary.

At times, social pressure or special situations may make it difficult to adhere to the diet; in those cases I suggest that the A temporarily backslide and eat the food available—picking those dishes that he feels will be least harmful and most nutritious. Creating guilt or mental anguish over a diet can be more harmful to the body than eating poor quality foods.

The process of adapting to a vegetarian diet should be as follows: first eliminate high-vibrational foods from the diet. Cut out beef and pork products, selecting the more easily digestible meats such as veal, lamb, chicken or fish. Over a period of time, eliminate veal and lamb, and eat only chicken, turkey or fish. Then work into eating only fish, and try reducing the intake of this protein to two or three times a week.

I suggest avoiding lobster, shrimp, mussels and clams; they are scavengers that live off the debris at the bottom of the ocean.

Except for their high iodine content, their nutritional value is of a poor quality. Tunafish and swordfish should also be strictly avoided as they have often been found to be contaminated with mercury, which is toxic. Purer fish such as cod, halibut, red snapper, salmon, haddock, sea bass and sea trout, all of which swim at a middle to upper level of the sea and have more nutrients, are preferable. Flounder and sole, considered "dirty fish" because they swim close to the surface and thrive on surface wastes, can be eaten, but should be done so only on occasion, such as once a week. As his body begins to balance and strengthen, animal proteins will no longer be necessary to the A, and fish, too, can be phased out of the diet. The A's protein will now be totally derived from vegetables and soy products such as tofu.

The A has a highly sensitive body and foods that are not harmonious to him may rapidly cause adverse reactions: headaches, nausea or pimples. During the change to vegetarianism, certain side effects may be experienced as the body purifies itself—throwing off years of accumulated toxicity caused by foods of poor quality and by foods inimical to his blood type. This is sometimes called the "healing crisis" and includes such reactions as headaches, diarrhea, nausea and fatigue. However, these conditions are usually only temporary and disappear as the body cleanses and balances itself.

The A is not a physically active person and therefore his nutritional needs are lower than those of people of other blood types. Once his body is in balance, he will not need vitamins because all his nutrients will come from vegetables, fruits and grains. However, during the initial stages of the diet, some low-dosage vitamins may be needed to strengthen debilitated organs or tissues. A full list of these vitamins is available in Chapter 8.

Since the A functions chiefly on nervous energy, it is important that he choose physical exercise which will have a calming effect. A Japanese study (independent of my work) has shown that most car accidents are caused by people with type-A blood. This does not surprise me because my own studies have shown that A's are usually jittery and on edge and, consequently, accident-prone.

Exercises such as jogging, calisthenics, gymnastics or contact sports have a stimulating effect on the A's body and will further excite him. Therefore, these activities should be done only with great restraint.

The A often feels he should work off his excessive nervous energy by strenuous exercise. When he does this, his immediate reaction is a feeling of well-being, but the stimulation can fatigue him and this aggravates his tension. The best exercises for the A are Hatha Yoga or T'ai Chi Ch'uan which will relax him, helping him to find a more normal level of energy. Light swimming or jogging, hiking, golfing and, on occasion, tennis are also beneficial.

The A should take lukewarm baths and showers for their calming effect. Hot baths and steam rooms, on the other hand, will drain the energy and should be taken only occasionally. Cold baths or showers will overstimulate the A.

My experience has shown that both the body and the mind are affected by colors (see Chapter 11), and I have found that the A should wear blues and greens, which will be soothing. These colors should also be used in decorating living quarters. Soft pastels such as beige, peach, rose or powder blue will also have a quieting effect on the A.

Let me tell you about one of my patients in order to show you how the principles I have outlined affect a specific person. A woman with type-A blood, who was in her middle fifties when she consulted me, had a chronic case of bronchial asthma. She had been following what she had believed to be the ideal diet all her life: meat, dairy products and vegetables. However, as I have discovered, the A cannot readily assimilate meats and dairy products and this diet caused her to form an excessive amount of catarrh.

Like most people with this condition, she had resorted to nasal sprays and antihistamines to relieve her and had used these medications for over twenty years, suppressing her symptoms— but worsening her condition.

I immediately set her on the way to health by curtailing her consumption of meat and dairy products and putting her on a strict vegetarian diet.

Her typical breakfast included such foods as oatmeal and soy milk and one slice of soy bread. For lunch, she had a mixed raw salad of greens, squash, sprouts, Jerusalem artichoke and cucumber. She was warned against eating tomatoes, which are highly acidic, and carrots, which are irritating to the A's stomach. For dinner, she ate another raw salad, a variety of steamed vegetables including asparagus, broccoli, okra, squash, fennel and string beans, and a serving of brown rice. To maintain her strength until she was adjusted to the vegetarian regimen, I prescribed fish twice a week. For protein, she ate tofu at every meal. Acidic grains such as buckwheat, millet and bulghur, which are harmful for the A, were not included in her diet.

Her vitamin program included one B-complex formula, 250 IU of Vitamin E, 10,000 IU of Vitamin A and 400 IU of Vitamin D daily. In addition, she took 500 mgs of Vitamin C every other day to help repair the tissue in her respiratory tract and raise her body's resistance against disease. She drank an herbal tea of Solomon's Seal throughout the day to soothe her and to cleanse the mucus from her chest. On this regimen, the patient attained her ideal, balanced health.

TYPE O

A person with type-O blood, or the "O," usually has a strong, well-developed physique, and is very physically active. The O's need for a vigorous physical life-style is as important to his well-being as is his diet. Because the O has a high-vibrational body, his main source or nourishment should be derived from foods high in protein: the O is definitely a meat-eater and I do *not* recommend that he try to be a vegetarian. He should eat such high-protein foods as calf's liver, chicken, lamb, turkey or fish daily.

When selecting his meats, the O should be aware that commercially bred cattle, lamb and pigs are no longer free-grazing animals. The majority of store-bought meats are from animals raised in pens, and injected with antibiotics and stilbestrol (a cancer-causing agent) to fatten them. Pork products should definitely be avoided for they are high in fat and low in nutrients. If beef can be obtained from pastured cattle that have not been artificially fattened, the O should eat the internal organs— kidneys, lungs, liver and heart—because they are excellent sources of protein. Muscle meats should be avoided because uric acid lodges in these tissues and when eaten, these meats can increase body toxicity. As with beef, lamb should also come from a free-grazing animal; however, as lamb is fatty, I recommend eating it only once a week.

Dairy products such as milk, yogurt and eggs are not as mucus-forming to the O as they are to the A and can be eaten as good supplementary sources of protein. It is preferable that milk products be made from raw and not commercial milk. During pasteurization, the enzyme phosphatase in milk, required for the assimilation of calcium, is destroyed. Cows used for raw-milk products are fed a better quality of food than those used in commercial products, are not restricted to the feed lot, and are under stricter supervision. I have seen recent tests showing that these animals have a lower bacterial count than conventional milk cows.

Whole-wheat products are not so acid-forming for the O as they are for the A. Therefore such grains as millet, buckwheat, barley and bran and pasta and whole-wheat bread can be eaten as desired. The O should also eat grains and breads made from soy beans to help balance the acid-alkaline level of his blood.

Some of the vegetables the O may select include: chick peas, leafy greens, celery, collards, cucumber, potatoes, corn, okra, broccoli, fennel, asparagus, sprouts, beans, squash, daikon, radishes, artichokes, carrots and mushrooms. The O may also eat tomatoes, which are only slightly acidic in his body; avocados, lentils, cabbage (white, red and savoy), green pepper, mustard greens, eggplant and turnips.

The recommended fruits for him are apples, oranges, mangoes, tangerines, peaches, grapes (black and green), Bing cherries, pineapples, strawberries, blueberries, cantaloupe, grapefruits, figs and only occasionally bananas, which have a very high fructose (fruit sugar) content.

Unlike the A, the O cannot derive all his nutrient requirements from his foods and will always require vitamin supplements. His dosages should be higher than the A's—provided he is involved in a vigorous exercise program or has a physically demanding occupation. If the O is inactive, or does not exercise regularly, dosage levels should be reduced because excess nutrients will not be utilized and burned off, and can become toxic.

As I said earlier, a demanding physical program is as important to the O as his diet. Although the O tends to be a muscular person, my studies have shown that his blood flow is naturally sluggish. Without a vigorous exercise program to activate his blood and energy, he can become lazy and lethargic. The more the O exercises, the more his body will be stimulated, leading to a great feeling of well-being. Jogging, gymnastics, calisthenics, hiking, swimming and bicycling are preferred exercises for the O and should be done vigorously and on a regular basis (an hour or two a day).

In a test I did with athletes, I discovered that after several hours of active exercise, the O's were rarely fatigued. On the contrary, their bodies were charged with energy and they were able to partake in further activities. Athletes with type-A blood, however, were usually more exhausted following their exercises because the A's tended to use more mental or nervous energy in their performance and consequently experienced a greater general drain. After exercise, the A's had little desire to engage in further activities or to socialize.

Although the O is a more physically inclined person than the A, this does not preclude his attaining a high level of intelligence or creativity. O's, however, seem to have more acquired, worldly wisdom than the A, who is often more instinctively clever.

Because the key to the O's well-being is the stimulation of his energy, hot and cold baths, cold showers and cold hip baths can be taken once or twice a day. Colors that will help to charge him up are reds, oranges, yellows and purples (see Chapter 11).

A good example of an O whose body was imbalanced because of improper diet is a young man who consulted me because, as he described himself, he was "worn out and mentally lackadaisical." He had been a vegetarian for five years, sustaining himself only on vegetables, fruits, seeds, yogurt and honey. On this diet, he had lost a considerable amount of weight and strength and had developed anemia (a deficiency of red corpuscles and hemoglobin in the blood).

In order to rebuild his body, I put him on a high-protein diet, similar to one recommended for a balanced O. He ate chicken, lamb and fish each once or twice a week, and I prescribed calf's liver twice weekly in order to increase his red-blood-cell count and cure his enervating anemia. He ate dairy products, fruits and such high-iron vegetables as kale, broccoli and carrots on a regular basis. Tofu was included in every meal, and at midday, he drank a high-protein milkshake made of raw milk, an egg, honey and protein powder. In addition, he munched on dried apricots during the day, which also introduced iron into his body.

To revitalize his body tissues, strengthen his nervous system and replenish his energy, I prescribed 50 mgs of vitamins B_1, B_2, and B_6 twice a day, plus 100 mgs of B_{12} four times a day. He drank ginseng tea twice a day to increase his physical energy.

As he recovered his health and strength, I reduced his intake of liver to once a week, and reduced the dried apricots (which are high in sugar as well as iron) to twice a week. Since he still desired to eat vegetarian meals one or two days a week, I suggested that he make those meals of two eggs, cottage cheese, four squares of tofu and a grain—such as millet, which is high in vegetable protein.

TYPE B

A person with type-B blood has a medial vibrational body, sharing the qualities and characteristics of both the O and A.

Constitutionally, he or she is stronger than the A, but less muscular than the O.

Not so intense in either body or mind as the O or A, the B is able to strike a better balance between his physical and mental pursuits: the B is the most centered or "grounded," the most physically and emotionally integrated of the three blood types. Whereas the A is a mental person, inclined to intellectual pursuits, and the O is driven by his need for physical activity, the B tends to cultivate his body and mind equally, developing a wide range of interests and abilities. It is not uncommon to find a B who excels in sports as well as in the intellectual arena or the arts; one who lives evenly in the spiritual and material worlds.

Because he has a middle-range vibrational body, the B can share in the dietary regimens of both the O and A. Meat and dairy products are not so mucus-forming to the B as they are to the A, and may be eaten. Since his body is not so active as the O's, his nutritional needs are not as great, and he does not need to eat meat everyday. An ideal diet for the B is meat—chicken, turkey, lamb or fish—three or four times a week, and a vegetarian regimen on the remaining days.

Similarly, the B can eat dairy products, which are slightly mucus-forming, and wheat products, which are only mildly acid-forming in his body, several times a week. The key to the B's diet is moderation. As long as he selects his food in moderation, his diet can be the broadest of all the blood types. He can share in both a vegetarian and animal-protein diet, and he has a wider variety of food to choose from than the A or AB.

For instance, the B can have wheatgerm, buckwheat, barley and whole wheat or seven or ten grain breads several times a week, balancing his diet on the other days with the alkaline soy products such as soy flakes, soy beans and soy bread. Cheese, such as ricotta or cottage cheese, can be eaten three times a week. He can have four eggs a week, and raw milk may be included in his cereal twice a week, soy milk five days a week. Brown rice, which is slightly acidic to the B, can be eaten twice a week. Legumes such as kidney, pinto and lima beans, which are high in starch and potentially constipating, should be eaten only once a week.

The vegetables the B may choose from include carrots, peas, string beans, celery, corn, okra, collards, asparagus, broccoli, kale, mushrooms, potatoes, watercress, leafy green endive and tomatoes. He can eat grapefruits, papaya, cantaloupe, strawberries, blueberries, peaches and apricots. The more acidic fruits such as apples, oranges, mangoes, and tangerines should be limited to once or twice a week, as should pears, which can create flatulence.

Like the O, the B cannot get all his nutritional requirements from his food and will need to take certain vitamin supplementation. However, his dosages should be low or medium potency, or determined by his physical activity or emotional states.

Exercise, which is not so vital to the B's regimen as it is to the A and O's, should also be done in moderation. Whereas the A is hyperstimulated and needs to be calmed, and the O is often sluggish and needing to be stimulated, the B's body is moderately charged. He can jog, hike, swim, or do gymnastics, calisthenics or Hatha Yoga for an hour to an hour-and-a-half several times a day. Whatever the exercise or sport, the B will find that he can simply enjoy himself, rather than work either to calm or to stimulate his body.

Warm baths and showers are best suited for the B, although cold or hot baths or saunas may be taken periodically and briefly, to help relax or invigorate him.

The B can choose his colors from a broad range of the spectrum, including reds and oranges to activate his body or mind, blues and greens to soothe his nerves, and mauves and violets to provide a mood conducive to reflection or meditation.

A typical case of a B with disorders caused by the wrong food for his blood type was that of a highly emotional college student who had taxed his kidneys and was suffering from oozing eczemic rashes.

As you have seen, the B is a middle-of-the-road blood type, and when he is not in a balanced state of health, he will react either like the O deprived of protein and become fatigued, or like the A, who produces an excessive amount of mucus on the wrong diet.

This young man's body had become clogged with wastes and mucus and he had to drastically reduce his intake of meats and dairy products to prevent the production of more catarrh.

This B could not have been able to sustain himself on the strict vegetarian diet appropriate to an A, so I recommended that he eat fish three times a week. I did not advise chicken, liver or lamb because these meats have a higher uric acid content, which would irritate his kidneys. To further aid kidney function, I had him eat asparagus and dandelion leaves every day, because they are the premiere kidney purifiers, in my experience.

I wished to prevent the increase of acidity in his body so I substituted alkaline products for whole-wheat grains. Grapefruit and watermelons were recommended for the young man to assist in the purification of his blood. I forbade all spices and condiments during this period because they can irritate the kidneys and bladder.

I recommended a daily dosage of the following vitamins: 50 mg vitamin B_6, 250 mg B_{12}, 10,000 IU vitamin A, 1,000 mg vitamin C, 400 mg vitamin D, and one low-potency B-complex formula. In addition, I prescribed dandelion tea and ten glasses of water a day to help flush the impurities from his blood and kidneys.

The student's mother, who was a nurse, asked me why I never gave her son a cortisone salve for his itching and oozing rashes. Cortisone is sometimes prescribed by medical doctors for eczema and other skin problems, but this drug only suppresses the inflammation without curing the underlying disease. The patient often seems to improve while an infection, for example, continues to progress.

To relieve the itching, I prescribed, instead of this very dangerous drug, a proven Natural remedy: oatmeal baths and packs. The "milk" of oatmeal immediately takes the sting out of a rash and by not suppressing the rash, allows it to heal. As the

50

student's kidneys strengthened and the toxicity was discharged from his body, all of his eczemic blotches vanished.

TYPE AB

People with type-AB blood (the "AB's") are similar in physical and mental characteristics to the A's. Like the A, the AB has a sensitive body and a naturally acute mind. When in a balanced condition, the AB, like the A, has a more active mind than body. However, the AB tends to be slightly stronger and more active than the A, and though his main source of nourishment should also come from the vegetable kingdom, the AB should fortify his body with an easily digestible protein, such as fish, once or twice a week.

Meats and dairy products are mucus-forming to the AB and should be avoided. Whole-wheat products are highly acid-forming in his body, and so soy-derived products should be eaten instead.

The diet of the AB is quite similar to that of the A. Some of the vegetables the AB can include in his diet are leafy greens such as: lettuce, beet greens, collards, Swiss chard and kale; watercress, asparagus, broccoli, carrots (boiled or steamed), fennel, okra, cucumbers, celery, squash, beans and potatoes. Tomatoes are too acidic for the AB and should be avoided or eaten sparingly. Avocados, which are rich in oil, should be eaten only occasionally, if at all. The AB should avoid cabbage, which causes excessive gas, and lentils, which are difficult to digest and too high a concentration of iron for his body.

The fruits he can choose include: papaya, strawberries, blueberries, gooseberries, grapefruits, cantaloupe, honeydew, peaches, apricots, dark plums, Bing cherries, watermelon and dark grapes.

In switching over to a vegetarian diet, as in all dietary change, the AB should proceed slowly. Beef and pork products should be eliminated first, and he should switch to the more easily digestible proteins in lamb, chicken, turkey and fish. After a period of time, he should eliminate lamb, and eat chicken, turkey and fish, and then eventually eliminate chicken and turkey until his animal-protein requirement is satisfied by eating fish twice a week.

When selecting seafood, the AB should remember that lobster, shrimp, mussels and clams feed off the debris at the bottom of the ocean, and although they are high in iodine, are of a poor nutritional quality. Salmon, halibut, scrod, haddock, flounder and cod would be preferable. Tuna and swordfish should be strictly avoided as they have sometimes been contaminated with mercury.

Like the A, the AB may experience some reactions as he changes to a vegetarian diet. Nausea, cramps, headaches and skin eruptions sometimes occur during the change of diet, but the AB should remember that these are only temporary conditions caused by the body's efforts to cleanse itself of toxicity, and not internal disorders.

Because his nutritional needs are low compared to the O or B, the AB will not require vitamins once his system is balanced. All his vitamins and minerals will come from his food. During the balancing stages, however, certain vitamins such as B_{12} or B_6 may be needed to help strengthen his body. Mega-vitamin therapy should be strictly avoided by the AB, because high dosages of vitamins may stress his body. *All* his vitamins should be of a low potency.

Because most AB's are slightly tense individuals, they function primarily on a nervous, kinetic energy. Therefore, the AB should do exercises that will calm and relax his body, not overstimulate it. Hatha Yoga and T'ai Chi Ch'uan are ideal for this. If the AB jogs, swims, hikes, or engages in competitive sports, he should try to pace himself and expend his energy economically, taking care that he neither excite nor tax his body.

Lukewarm showers and baths are best for the AB. I have found that the most soothing colors for him are blue and green.

A factor that I always take into consideration when I create a diet that will harmonize food to the vibrational body of each blood type is the balance between each individual's input of food and his exertion of physical energy.

For example, although O's are usually very active, there are some O's who tend to be sedentary and therefore have less need for a high-protein diet than do the more active representatives of the blood type. The sedentary O should reduce his intake of meat and dairy products to his energy needs—from every day to only four times a week or so. Excessive protein can actually harm the body by creating a surplus of energy which, by making the body's systems work harder, can stress and debilitate them.

Similarly, an A or AB with a physically demanding occupation, such as a construction worker or professional athlete, may not be able to meet his energy requirements on a vegetarian regimen. This atypically active A or AB may have to supplement his diet with chicken, turkey or fish. As he is very active, his body will burn off the nutrients that a more sedentary A or AB would not be able to assimilate.

Since I have been working with blood types, I have come across very few people who had a real intuitive sense of the foods that they required. Most of my patients, who had eaten to satisfy their taste buds, have accumulated high levels of toxicity and weakened their bodies. I could never recommend a diet based on a balanced state of health for these patients, and so I adapt a diet from the ideal state according to each patient's current physical condition.

Healing though nutrition is dynamic and ever-changing. A diet that I designed for you today in your current state of less-than-perfect well-being may no longer be right for you when, in the future, your body heals and achieves a state of balance. Diets have to be augmented, adding more foods to meet new physical needs, or reduced when certain foods are no longer required for their nutrient value.

Following are my recommended diets for each blood type in a perfectly balanced state of health. These diets are the ideal—the reality must be adjusted to each individual. Later I am going to show you how you can, by evaluating your current state of well-being and vitality, create a diet that will help you to achieve the state of health and energy you long for.

THE DIETS

Type A: Vegetarian
No meats, dairy, whole-wheat products.

VEGETABLES:
Asparagus, agar, alfalfa, artichokes, bamboo sprouts, beets and beet greens, bean sprouts—all types, broccoli, beans (pinto, kidney, soy, string, etc.), chicory, celery, boiled carrots, white corn, collards, cucumber, dandelion greens, daikon, endive, escarole, fennel, kale, kohlrabi, all lettuces (iceberg, romaine, red leaf, Boston, etc.), lentils (once a month), mushrooms, okra, parsley, white or sweet potato (baked), rugola (arugola), seaweed, Swiss chard, all types of squash, spinach (once every two months), watercress, zucchini.

FRUITS:
Apricot, blackberries, blueberries, Bing cherries, cantaloupe, elderberries, grapefruit, lime, lemon, plums (dark Italian), papaya, peach, raspberries, strawberries, watermelon, dates, raisins, currants and pears (once a month).

JUICES:
Grapefruit, diluted papaya, water and lemon.

GRAINS AND CEREALS:
Rolled oats, cornmeal, brown rice, soy flakes, soy granules.

BREADS:
Soy loafs, sprouted wheat.

SPICES AND CONDIMENTS:
Oregano, garlic, tarragon, thyme, rosemary, basil, kelp powder, parsley and seasalt.

OILS:
Sunflower, safflower, sesame, soy and olive.

MARGARINES:
Soy, safflower, lecithin.

54

HERBAL TEAS:
Chamomile, dandelion, peppermint, rose hip, rosemary.

Type O: High Animal Protein

MEATS:
Veal, lamb, chicken, turkey, calf's liver, kidney and lung.

FISH:
Sea trout, sea bass, haddock, halibut, flounder, bluefish, red snapper, whiting, salmon, cod, scrod, brook trout, sole.

DAIRY PRODUCTS:
Raw cow's milk, goat's milk, soybean milk, yogurt, sweet butter, farmer's cheese, ricotta, cottage cheese, mozzarella cheese; four to five eggs a week.

MARGARINES:
Soy, lecithin, safflower.

WHOLE-GRAIN PRODUCTS:
Barley, millet, wheat grains, pilaf, buckwheat, pasta.

VEGETABLES:
Asparagus, avocado, agar, alfalfa, artichokes, bamboo sprouts, beets and beet greens, bean sprouts (all types), broccoli, beans (all types), white and savoy cabbages, chick peas, chicory, celery, cucumber, carrots, white corn, dandelion greens, daikon, eggplant, endive, escarole, fennel, kale, kelp, kohlrabi, lettuce (all types), lentils, leeks, mustard greens, mushrooms, okra, olives, onions, fresh peas, green pepper, parsley, baked white and sweet potatoes, radishes, rugola, rhubarb, seaweed, Swiss chard, squash (all types), spinach (once a month), snow-pea pods, watercress, water chestnuts, yeast, tomatoes, turnips, and zucchini.

FRUITS:
Apples, apricots, blackberries, blueberries, Bing cherries, bananas (once a month), cantaloupe, elderberries, figs, guava, grapefruit, black grapes,

honeydew melon, limes, lemons, mangoes, oranges, pomegranate, plums (dark Italian), papaya, pineapple, peach, pear, raspberries, strawberries, tangerine, watermelon, dates, raisins, currants (occasionally).

JUICES:
Apple, grapefruit, orange, papaya, water and lemon, carrot (occasionally).

CEREALS:
Shredded wheat, wheat germ, soya/wheat, oatmeal, cornmeal, bran, soy flakes, soy granules.

BREADS:
Whole-wheat, buckwheat, seven or ten grain, Scandinavian crispbreads, rye, soy loaf, sprouted wheat.

SPICES AND CONDIMENTS:
Tarragon, oregano, garlic, cloves, onion, thyme, scallions, rosemary, basil, seasalt, parsley, garlic, kelp powder, apple-cider vinegar.

OILS:
Sunflower, soy, safflower, sesame, peanut and olive.

HERBAL TEAS:
Chamomile, dandelion, peppermint, rose hip, rosemary, parsley, ginseng.

Type B: Animal-Protein/Vegetarian

MEATS:
Veal, lamb, chicken, turkey.

FISH:
Sea trout, brook trout, sea bass, haddock, flounder, halibut, bluefish, red snapper, whiting, salmon, cod, scrod, sole.

DAIRY PRODUCTS:
Skimmed milk, soybean milk, yogurt, sweet butter, three or four eggs a week, farmer's, ricotta, and cottage cheeses.

MARGARINES:
Soy, lecithin, safflower.

OILS:
Sunflower, safflower, sesame, soy, olive.

WHOLE-GRAIN PRODUCTS:
Barley, millet, buckwheat, wheat grains, pilaf, pasta.

VEGETABLES:
Asparagus, agar, alfalfa, artichokes, bamboo sprouts, beets and beet greens, bean sprouts (all types), broccoli, beans (all types), white cabbage (occasionally), chicory, celery, cucumber, boiled carrots, raw carrots (occasionally), white corn, collards, dandelion greens, daikon, eggplant, endive, escarole, kale, kelp, kohlrabi, lettuce (all types), lentils (occasionally), mushrooms, okra, fresh peas, parsley, baked white and sweet potato, pumpkin, rugola, seaweed, Swiss chard, squash (all types), spinach (once a month), snow-pea pods, tomatoes (once every two weeks), watercress, water chestnuts, zucchini (once a week).

FRUITS:
Apple (once a week), apricot, blackberries, blueberries, Bing cherries, cantaloupe, elderberry, grapefruit, honeydew, lime, lemon, oranges, plums (dark Italian), peach, pear (once a week), raspberries, strawberries, tangerine, watermelon. Dates, figs, currants and raisins occasionally.

JUICES:
Apple (once a week), grapefruit, orange (several times a week), papaya, water and lemon.

CEREALS:
Shredded wheat, wheatgerm, soya/wheat, oatmeal, cornmeal, bran, soy flakes, soy granules.

BREADS:
Whole-wheat, buckwheat, seven or ten grain, soy loafs, sprouted wheat, Scandinavian crispbreads.

SPICES AND CONDIMENTS:
Tarragon, cloves, oregano, garlic, thyme, rosemary, basil, parsley, kelp powder, apple-cider vinegar (several times a week).

HERBAL TEAS:
Chamomile, peppermint, dandelion, rose hip, rosemary, ginseng, parsley.

Type AB: Vegetarian/Fish
No meats, dairy or whole-wheat products.

FISH:
Sea trout, sea bass, haddock, flounder, halibut, salmon, cod, scrod, sole (any of these once or twice a week).

VEGETABLES:
Asparagus, agar, alfalfa, artichokes, bamboo sprouts, beets and beet greens, bean sprouts (all types), broccoli, beans (all types), chicory, celery, boiled carrots, corn, collards, cucumber, dandelion greens, daikon, endive, escarole, fennel, kale, kohlrabi, lettuce (all types), lentils (once a month), mushrooms, okra, fresh peas, parsley, baked white or sweet potato, rugola, seaweed, Swiss chard, squash (all types), spinach (once every two months), watercress, zucchini.

FRUITS:
Apricot, blackberries, blueberries, Bing cherries, cantaloupe, elderberries, grapefruit, lime, lemon, plums (dark Italian), papaya, peach, raspberries, strawberries, watermelon. Figs, raisins, currants and dates (once a month).

JUICES:
Grapefruit, diluted papaya, water and lemon.

GRAINS AND CEREALS:
Rolled oats, cornmeal, brown rice, soy flakes, soy granules.

58

BREADS:
Soy loafs, sprouted wheat.

SPICES AND CONDIMENTS:
Oregano, garlic, tarragon, thyme, rosemary, basil, kelp powder, parsley and seasalt.

OILS:
Sunflower, safflower, sesame, soy and olive.

MARGARINES:
Soy, safflower and lecithin.

HERBAL TEAS:
Chamomile, dandelion, peppermint, rose hip, rosemary.

Many patients come to me because they want to lose weight without becoming enervated or lowering their body's resistance to disease. Although normalization of weight will almost invariably occur when you follow the proper diet for your blood type and energy requirements, sometimes weight reduction may be vital to a patient's health.

No one weight reduction program is correct for everyone. However, my program is based on your blood type and it will respect your individuality and the particular needs of your body. It will help you to control your weight without damaging your system, now or in the future.

In certain instances, my suggestions for this diet may seem to contradict the guidelines I have previously set down for the ideal types. For example, on the weight-reduction diet, it is permissible to eat fruit with vegetables and bread with eggs. These exceptions are allowed because weight-reduction diets are very demanding and, during the short amount of time you will follow this diet, the usually forbidden combinations of food will not harm you.

APPROACH TO A HEALTHFUL WEIGHT-REDUCTION PROGRAM

1. Remain on diet for about one month. Take the vitamins recommended in this book. Consult your physician.

2. If possible, limit bread consumption to one or two slices a day. Do not use sugar. Equally, avoid saccharin or any other sugar substitutes, as they have produced cancer in laboratory animals. Onions, which are rich in sugar, and alcoholic beverages, which also have a high sugar content and absorb the B-complex vitamins in the body, should not be consumed. In addition, refrain from eating potatoes, noodles and other flour-based foods.

3. The quantity of meat intake (where applicable) is left to your discretion. However, since you are trying to decrease the amount of food you eat and thereby reduce the size of your stomach, steadily reduce the size of your helpings.

4. Rotate these herbal teas routinely: chickweed (to assist in the elimination of water); dandelion (to cleanse the kidneys and liver); peppermint (to soothe the stomach); and chamomile (to relax the stomach and the rest of the body). Although black coffee is allowed during the program, it is preferable that you eliminate it in favor of the teas.

5. Each morning upon rising, squeeze one-half a lemon into a tall glass of purified water and drink it at least ten minutes before eating breakfast.

This program may seem more difficult to adhere to than many other programs you have undoubtedly come across, but I assure you that by following this diet, you will both lose weight and maintain a satisfactory energy level.

TYPE A AND TYPE AB

SUNDAY

BREAKFAST
½ cantaloupe
1 slice toasted soya bread
1 cup herbal tea

LUNCH
Salad: Lettuce, tomato, celery, watercress, cucumber, beansprouts
1 slice toasted soya bread
Dressing: Safflower oil, Lemon juice
Beverage: 1 cup herbal tea

MONDAY

BREAKFAST
½ grapefruit
1 slice toasted soya bread
1 cup herbal tea

LUNCH
Salad: Lettuce, stalk of celery, one tomato, ½ square tofu, parsley
Dressing: Safflower oil, Lemon juice
Beverage: 1 cup herbal tea

TUESDAY

BREAKFAST
½ grapefruit
1 slice toasted soya bread
1 cup herbal tea

LUNCH
Salad: Sections of 1 grapefruit and 1 orange on a bed of lettuce
Beverage: 1 cup herbal tea

WEDNESDAY

BREAKFAST
½ grapefruit
1 slice toasted soya bread
1 cup herbal tea

LUNCH
Salad: ½ head of lettuce
1 can of water-packed sardines
1 slice toasted soya bread
Beverage: 1 cup herbal tea

THURSDAY

BREAKFAST
½ grapefruit
1 slice toasted soya bread
1 cup herbal tea

LUNCH
Salad: Lettuce
Dressing: Safflower oil, Lemon juice
2 eggs poached
1 slice toasted soya bread
Beverage: 1 cup herbal tea

FRIDAY

BREAKFAST
½ grapefruit
1 slice toasted soya bread
1 cup herbal tea

LUNCH
Salad: Lettuce, cucumbers, watercress, beansprouts, celery, tomato, ½ square tofu, parsley
Dressing: Safflower oil, Lemon juice
Beverage: 1 cup herbal tea

SATURDAY

BREAKFAST
½ grapefruit
1 slice toasted soya bread
1 cup herbal tea

LUNCH
Salad: Sections of 1 grapefruit and 1 orange on a bed of lettuce
1 slice toasted soya bread
Beverage 1 cup herbal tea

DINNER
1/4 chicken, skin removed, boiled or broiled
Vegetables (steamed only): Swiss chard, dandelion, asparagus
Salad:
Lettuce, cucumber, celery, beansprouts, tomato
1/2 square tofu
Dressing:
Safflower oil
Lemon juice
Beverage:
1 cup herbal tea

DINNER
1 salmon steak broiled
Vegetables (steamed only): Kale, string beans, broccoli tips
Salad:
Lettuce, tomato, sprouts
Dressing:
Safflower oil
Lemon juice
1 slice toasted soya bread
Beverage:
1 cup herbal tea

DINNER
1/4 chicken, skin removed, boiled or broiled
Vegetables (steamed only): Dandelion, broccoli tips, asparagus
Salad:
Lettuce, cucumber, celery, parsley
Dressing:
Safflower oil
Lemon juice
1 slice soya toast
Beverage:
1 cup herbal tea

DINNER
1/2 grapefruit
Salad:
Lettuce, celery, tomato, cucumber, parsley, spinach, chicory, raw fresh mushrooms
1/2 square tofu
Dressing:
Safflower oil
Lemon juice
Beverage:
1 cup herbal tea

DINNER
1/2 lb. flounder, broiled
Vegetables: (steamed only) String beans
Salad:
Lettuce, beansprouts, celery and cucumbers
Dressing:
Safflower oil
Lemon juice
Beverage:
1 cup herbal tea

DINNER
Vegetables (steamed only): Kale, kelp, okra, Swiss chard, snow-pea pods
Salad:
Lettuce, celery, chicory, watercress, beansprouts, parsley
Dressing:
Safflower oil
Lemon juice
1 slice soya toast
Beverage:
1 cup herbal tea

DINNER
1/2 lb. haddock
Salad:
Lettuce, tomato, chicory, celery, beansprouts, cucumber, parsley
Dressing:
Safflower oil
Lemon juice
Beverage:
1 cup herbal tea

When eating fruit before a meal, always wait ten minutes before eating the rest of the food.

TYPE O

	SUNDAY	MONDAY	TUESDAY	WEDNESDAY	THURSDAY	FRIDAY	SATURDAY
BREAKFAST	½ grapefruit 2 poached eggs 1 slice whole-wheat toast 1 cup herbal tea	½ grapefruit 1 slice whole-wheat bread toasted 1 cup herbal tea	½ grapefruit 1 slice whole-wheat bread toasted 1 cup herbal tea	½ grapefruit 1 slice whole-wheat bread toasted 1 cup herbal tea	½ grapefruit 1 slice whole-wheat bread toasted 1 cup herbal tea	½ grapefruit 1 slice whole-wheat bread toasted 1 cup herbal tea	½ grapefruit 1 slice whole-wheat bread toasted 1 cup herbal tea
LUNCH	½ cantaloupe 4 oz cottage cheese Lettuce, beansprouts, chicory, celery ¼ square tofu *Dressing:* Safflower oil/lemon 1 cup herbal tea	4 oz salt-free cottage cheese Wedges of tomato 1 slice whole-wheat toast 1 cup herbal tea	Wedges of lettuce ½ papaya 1 cup herbal tea	½ cantaloupe 4 oz cottage cheese, lettuce 1 cup herbal tea	Wedges of lettuce ½ papaya 1 cup herbal tea	8 oz plain yogurt with 2 tbsp. wheat-germ 1 cup herbal tea	*Salad:* Lettuce, cucumbers, bean-sprouts, tomato *Dressing:* Safflower oil Lemon juice 1 cup herbal tea

DINNER
¼ lb. steak, lean, broiled
Salad:
Cucumbers and beansprouts
Dressing:
Safflower/lemon
Vegetables:
Steamed kale, Swiss chard, broccoli, dandelion
Beverage:
1 cup herbal tea

DINNER
2 lean lamb chops
Salad:
Lettuce, beansprouts, chicory
Dressing:
Safflower oil lemon juice
Beverage:
1 cup herbal tea

DINNER
½ grapefruit
¼ chicken, skin removed, broiled, baked, boiled
Vegetables:
Steamed broccoli, asparagus, string beans
Salad:
Lettuce, cucumbers, sprouts
Dressing:
Safflower oil/lemon
Beverage:
1 cup herbal tea

DINNER
Salmon steak baked/broiled
Salad:
Watercress, tomato, mushrooms, chicory, celery, kale, beansprouts
Dressing:
Safflower/lemon
1 slice whole-wheat toast
Beverage:
1 cup herbal tea

DINNER
1 veal chop, lean, broiled
Salad:
Spinach with mushrooms
Dressing:
Safflower/lemon
Vegetables:
Steamed beet leaves, dandelion, asparagus
1 slice whole-wheat toast
Beverage:
1 cup herbal tea

DINNER
1 flounder fillet baked/broiled
Salad:
Lettuce, cucumbers, beansprouts, ¼ square tofu
Dressing:
Safflower/lemon
Vegetables:
Steamed broccoli
1 slice whole-wheat toast
1 cup herbal tea

DINNER
½ grapefruit
½ chicken, skin removed, baked, boiled, broiled
Salad:
Lettuce, celery, cucumbers, beansprouts
Dressing:
Safflower/lemon
Vegetables:
Steamed spinach, escarole, broccoli, kale
½ slice whole-wheat toast
Beverage:
1 cup herbal tea

Late night snack: either 1 apple of ½ grapefruit. When eating fruit before a meal, always wait ten minutes before eating the rest of the food.

TYPE B

	SUNDAY	MONDAY	TUESDAY	WEDNESDAY	THURSDAY	FRIDAY	SATURDAY
BREAKFAST	½ grapefruit 1 slice toasted soya bread 1 cup herbal tea	½ grapefruit 1 slice toasted soya bread 1 cup herbal tea	½ grapefruit 1 slice toasted whole–wheat bread 1 cup herbal tea	½ grapefruit 1 slice toasted soya bread 1 cup herbal tea	½ grapefruit 1 slice toasted whole–wheat bread 1 cup herbal tea	½ grapefruit 1 slice toasted soya bread 1 cup herbal tea	½ grapefruit 1 slice toasted whole–wheat bread 1 cup herbal tea
LUNCH	½ grapefruit 1 orange on bed of lettuce 1 slice toasted soya bread *Beverage:* 1 cup herbal tea	*Salad:* Lettuce, tomato, beansprouts, celery, cucumber, chicory, parsley *Dressing:* Safflower oil/lemon ½ square tofu 1 slice soya bread toasted *Beverage:* 1 cup herbal tea	½ grapefruit 1 orange on bed of lettuce 1 slice whole–wheat bread toasted *Beverage:* 1 cup herbal tea	½ cantaloupe 8-oz cup of plain yogurt 1 slice toasted soya bread *Beverage:* 1 cup herbal tea	2 hard–boiled eggs 1 slice whole–wheat toast Lettuce *Beverage:* 1 cup herbal tea	*Salad:* Lettuce wedges ⅛ square tofu 1 slice toasted soya bread *Beverage:* 1 cup herbal tea	Spinach salad with fresh mushrooms ⅛ square tofu *Dressing:* Safflower oil/lemon *Beverage:* 1 cup herbal tea

DINNER
½ cantaloupe
¼ chicken, skin removed, broiled, baked or boiled
Vegetables: Steamed beet leaves, broccoli, kale
Salad: Cucumbers
Dressing: Safflower oil/lemon
Beverage: 1 cup herbal tea

DINNER
¼ chicken, skin removed, broiled
Vegetables (steamed): Beet leaves, dandelion, asparagus
Salad: Lettuce, beansprouts, cucumbers
Dressing: Safflower/lemon
Beverage: 1 cup herbal tea

DINNER
1 salmon steak baked
Salad: Lettuce, cucumbers, chicory, beansprouts
Dressing: Safflower oil/lemon
Vegetables: Steamed string beans, dandelion, broccoli tips
Beverage: 1 cup herbal tea

DINNER
Salad: Spinach, beet leaves, lettuce, chicory, mushrooms, tomato, beansprouts
½ square tofu
Vegetables (steamed): Asparagus, broccoli
Dressing: Safflower oil/lemon
Beverage: 1 cup herbal tea

DINNER
1 halibut steak
Vegetables: Steamed kale, escarole
Salad: Lettuce, cucumbers
Dressing: Safflower oil/lemon
Beverage: 1 cup herbal tea

DINNER
½ chicken, skin removed, broiled
Vegetables: Steamed broccoli, asparagus
Salad: Lettuce, ½ tomato, cucumbers, beansprouts
Dressing: Safflower oil/lemon
Beverage: 1 cup herbal tea

DINNER
½ lb. veal chops, lean, broiled
Vegetables: Steamed kale, asparagus
Salad: Lettuce, tomato, celery, watercress, beansprouts
Dressing: Safflower oil/lemon
Beverage: 1 cup herbal tea

When eating fruit before a meal, always wait ten minutes before you continue eating the rest of the food.
Night snack: Apple once a week. Remainder of days ½ grapefruit.

5

How I Create
a Health Care Program

I believe that healing should be a creative act and that each treatment should be unique, designed especially for the patient in his current state of health.

After examining a patient and diagnosing his condition through the study of his eyes, I then determine his blood type. Then, I create a cure in harmony with his needs. This is a step-by-step process that includes rebuilding his lost strengths, undoing acquired susceptibilities fostered through improper diet or stress, and gradually revitalizing his energy to bring him back to a state of health. My program has three parts: a general introduction to nutrition and health care; an individualization of the ideal blood-type diet; and the creation of a specific regimen for the patient's current physical condition.

One of the first things I tell a patient is that his body can be compared to the actor or singer who struggles for years to become what is termed "an overnight success" by the press. Health, like success, is determined by a long pursuit: eating. However, the "overnight" result of ten to twenty years of improper and excessive eating is not success but ill health—perhaps high blood pressure, a heart attack, or arthritic pain.

The very first thing I make clear to the patient is that his years of irresponsible eating and perhaps immoderate drinking and smoking have caused toxicity in his body and eroded his health. Once the responsibility for health has been put where it belongs— in the patient's own hands—I tell him that given the right conditions, illness and physical decay can be reversed and healthy and youthful vitality rejuvenated.

But this depends solely upon how much effort the person wants to make. It's not always true that a person's desire for health is equaled by his determination to regain it. Many people think that it's going to be recovered by wishing on a star. To help my patients get an idea of what they can expect from their efforts, I ask them two questions (you may want to think about them before embarking on your own natural cure): How much health do you want returned? How much of your current life-style and eating habits are you willing to change to regenerate your well-being?

Most of my patients give the same answers: they want all their health and they want it NOW. Some have demanded it of me, as if I took it away from them and with some magic potion can give it back. If it were that simple I would. But there are no overnight, instant cures in Natural Healing, no drugs to temporarily relieve an ache or subdue a symptom.

Nature has inviolate laws; and just as it has taken time to lose the gift of health given you at birth, it's going to take a period of time and a certain amount of determination on your part to get it back. I always tell my patients that ultimately your desire for health will be the measure of health returned to you.

These principles explained, I begin with step one of the program—a general introduction to nutrition and health care—by recommending that the person examine the kinds of foods he is currently eating. It would be a good idea if you did the same. Make a list of all the foods you include in your daily meals. The foods most often mentioned by my patients are pizza, hamburgers, fried foods, coffee, sugar, white bread, cupcakes, Coca-Cola and such convenience items as TV dinners. How about you?

This, I always find extraordinary. No matter how many times I hear it, it never ceases to amaze me just how large a part of the American diet these foods comprise; even though their harmful effects on the body have been dramatized over and over again. Not only in health books, but in daily papers, magazines, radio and television. Not just by nutritionists and health nuts, but by esteemed doctors, professors and such government agencies as the FDA and the Department of Agriculture.

We hear, for instance, that every year the average American consumes approximately one hundred and fifty pounds of refined sugar—that's about thirty-five teaspoons per day—even though it is practically common knowledge that sugar is stripped of its nutrient qualities during the refining process and is hazardous to teeth, mental health and the body's metabolism. The very same American also eats meats preserved with such dangerous chemicals as sodium nitrite, which is used to control botulism at the risk of causing cancer; canned foods packed with BTA, a petroleum product banned in Europe because it is suspected of being carcinogenic; and vegetables sprayed with poisonous pesticides.

With what results? The inevitable results are exemplified by a 1976 study sponsored by the U.S. Office of Education, which shows a decline in the health and physical fitness of the most recent generation of American boys and girls who were raised on inferior synthesized foods. This reverses a one-hundred-year trend of increasing health! A recent report from the Center for Science in the Public Interest, a consumer organization, entitled "The Changing American Diet," reveals that one of the prime reasons for this shift in national well-being has been directly linked to the 50-percent increase in the use of processed foods containing sugar in the American diet since the turn of the century.

So as a first step in a patient's health program, I advise him to become *aware* of the foods he is now eating. I advise him to read labels and study ingredients. Discover which foods have sodium nitrite, artificial coloring, BTA and other preservatives. I suggest that he buy books and learn what effects the foods he is eating can have on his body. Once he has done his research and realized the potential harm he is doing to himself, his desire to help himself usually increases dramatically.

Now that he has a new awareness, I then suggest that he eliminate as many processed and refined foods as possible—but gradually. I emphasize that a person should make these changes over a period of weeks, and at a relaxed pace, unless his condition is severe and requires drastic measures. Changing one's eating habits can be very unsettling even for people who are eager to help themselves.

If a person is a "sugar addict" I advise him to cut down on high-sugar foods such as chocolate bars. If he is now eating one or two a day, I recommend cutting back to one every other day, and then one every third day. Eventually, as a means of satisfying his sugar hunger, I suggest substituting honey in hot beverages or eating snacks made with honey, which, though high in glucose (sugar), is a better quality food than refined or brown sugar.

If canned foods play a prominent part in his diet, I suggest that he switch to frozen foods or increase his intake of fresh fruits and vegetables, for canned foods are usually too rich in sugar, salt and preservatives. I encourage him to buy unsprayed organic fresh fruits and vegetables from a health food store. (Comparison shopping will show that inflation has put the price of commercial produce virtually on a par with organic foods.)

I recommend fertile, organic eggs, also available from a health food store. These eggs are from free-roaming hens that are fed a better grade of food, and have not been injected with antibiotics, which can be transmitted to the human bloodstream, bringing unnecessary toxins into the body. Other animal products such as cheese, butter, yogurt and milk should be from either certified raw cows' milk or goats' milk, because both are more nutritious than the equivalent products made from pasteurized cows' milk.

I also tell him to avoid beef and pork products because commercially raised steers are injected with agents that may cause cancer and are also laden with high amounts of toxic acids, and pork products have a high fat content and may harbor the trichinosis-causing worm.

If a patient or his family want meat in their diet, I recommend eating veal or lean lamb, for these meats come from younger animals whose bodies have not accumulated such a high degree of uric acid. If the person eats chicken or turkey, I suggest he buy it from the health food store or from a farmer who does not inject fowl with antibiotics or treat them with hormone pellets. If organic chickens are unavailable, I advise the person to buy the best grade commercial product and always discard the neck because hormone pellets are usually implanted in the neck area of the bird. I have known cases where a person's hormonal system was disrupted by the ingestion of such a pellet.

I also recommend that he select whole-wheat products, which are rich in B-complex vitamins and bulk, which the body needs for proper elimination. (Products made from refined or enriched flours have most of their vitamins and bulk processed out.) He should use only cold-pressed oils such as sunflower, safflower, sesame or olive oils, which have not been hydrogenated or subjected to intense heat destroying the beneficial fatty acids. I recommend baking or broiling food because frying greatly alters the chemical composition of food, increasing the anti-Vitamin A factor, which reduces this vitamin's availability and may cause such an effect as poor eyesight. I advise drinking bottled spring water or attaching a water filter to the faucet. Plain tap water may have a high concentration of airborne pollutants, chlorine (added at the reservoir to control bacteria), and in some areas of the country, cancer-causing radioactive particles or a certain amount of chemical or sewer seepage.

I advise the patient to avoid using certain types of utensils when preparing food. Aluminum pots and pans can cause indigestion or aluminum poisoning if the soft metal combines with the food during preparation. Although many health practitioners recommend stainless steel cookware, recent tests have shown that small amounts of chrome from the pots can be absorbed by the food, which over a period of time, can increase risk of heart disease. At high temperatures, Teflon-coated ware also emits toxic particles into food. Therefore, I recommend that the patient use cast iron, enameled or Pyrex ware, which have no toxic effect on food when cooking.

Since one of the common causes of many digestive disturbances is overeating, I recommend that the patient try to reduce the amount of food eaten at one meal. Most people gorge themselves. They stretch their stomachs three to four times its normal size, which forces the blood to rush to the abdominal area, resulting in a sudden lethargy. The best way to finish a meal is to leave the table with a slight hunger.

Cigarette smoking and drinking alcohol are two of the most difficult habits to change. Patients often tell me that wine and brandy aid the body in digestion. More often than not they have heard this tale from a representative of the liquor industry. Alcohol, in fact, robs the body of vitamins. However, if the patient wishes to drink, I recommend he give up hard liquor in favor of red or white wine. A spritzer, half white wine/half club soda is the drink I suggest.

Recent tests on cigarette smoking reveal that not only is it injurious to the smoker, the smoke also affects anyone in the smoker's immediate environment. After thirty minutes in a smoke-filled room, a nonsmoker has a higher than normal heart rate and blood pressure, and the carbon monoxide in his blood is sufficient to impair his ability to distinguish the brightness of lights from oncoming cars. A study of Erie County, Pennsylvania, married couples has shown that women who were nonsmokers but married to men who smoked became "passive smokers" and died an average of four to five years younger than nonsmoking women married to nonsmokers.

I never tell a patient to quit smoking all at once. Most smokers have tried to give up smoking one time or another and know that this technique is almost impossible. Instead, I recommend that the patient cut the amount of cigarettes he is smoking by about a quarter, then half, reducing as much as possible over a period of time. If a person has to smoke, I also suggest he does so only when he is alone.

I also recommend that a person reduce or eliminate such caffeine drinks as coffee or tea. Caffeine is a stimulant. Assimilated into the body in the quantity most Americans consume it—in two to ten cups of coffee a day—it can be harmful to the nervous system, unsettling to the mind, and have an aggravating effect on those with hypoglycemia. A half cup of coffee, taken black without milk, sugar or honey, several times a week, however, will not have an adverse effect, and in fact will act as a good diuretic stimulating the kidneys to increase urination. If a person experiences such undesirable reactions as dizziness or sudden lapses of energy after drinking coffee, however, I advise him to eliminate it from his diet immediately. The same goes for tea.

Many other factors can affect a person's health. I suggest that the patient examine his living conditions. What is the ecology of the area in which he lives? Does he live, for example, by a polluting factory? By a major highway? Is he exposed to any form of radiation where he works? Asbestos dust? Loud noises or bright flashing lights? I also suggest that he take stock of his clothing. Are his clothes cottons and woolens that allow air to flow through to the body? Or are they synthetics, which prevent the skin from breathing properly, clogging the pores, and inhibiting the perspiration of toxic wastes?

These are some of the many general changes I ask a patient to consider making at the beginning of the program. After several weeks at this level, I ask him to evaluate how he feels. The elimination of many "junk foods" can quickly cause an increase of energy and a heightened feeling of well-being. In some instances, people respond with such a surge of strength and vitality that they think they've recovered their total health. However, this is a "false high." If the person stayed at this diet level for any extended period of time, he would be relieved of minor body discomforts but would not undergo a significant healing and might even do damage to his body.

A young man in his twenties who had been trying to rid himself of an embarrassing case of post-adolescent acne by experimenting with all kinds of ointments and soaps, wrote me a letter saying that, "It's been only ten days since I stopped eating everything in sight and already many sores and blotches have disappeared." Because his elimination system had been sluggish and wastes had not been thoroughly evacuated from his body, he could have used those remedies the rest of his life without any significant changes. But, by reducing fried foods, butter and heavy meats and eating more fruits and vegetables, his digestive and elimination systems had quickly responded so that his body had begun to discharge many of the toxicities it had been retaining. When the wastes were eliminated through the proper channels, they no longer exuded from his skin nor caused eruptions on his face.

A woman, who for ten years had had constant diarrhea, discomfort after eating, gas and belching, and who had undergone "the whole gamut of exploratory tests," including barium enemas and rectal examinations, was told by her doctors that there was absolutely nothing they could find wrong with her. She was given antacids and various drugs for her stomach but without any positive results. After only one month of changing her diet, all her symptoms disappeared and she said, "I suddenly had a new life."

Although this first step can produce a new and wonderful feeling of vitality, I must emphasize that it is just the beginning. However, the patient must decide whether to take the next step and go deeper into the healing process to regain even more of his energy and well-being. I never push a person to continue. Because, in truth, I am not really doing the healing. I have actually never healed anyone in my entire life. All I do is make some suggestions; the real healing is done by Nature. If the patient agrees to continue to provide the conditions in which Nature can do Her work helping his body move toward its natural state, which is health, then we proceed to step two: a regimen individualized to his specific blood type.

In step two, I explain the concept of the ideal blood type: what a person in that state of health should normally eat and how the patient must gradually work toward the ideal. Here again, I ask the patient how much of his current life-style he is willing to change and how much health he wants to recover. I tell him that if he can discipline himself quickly without sustaining mental stress during the dietary change, he can make rapid progress in cleansing and strengthening his body.

But most people don't want to give up all their sweets or condiments, their late night parties and wine, so I suggest a compromise regimen which results in a slower, less dramatic recovery of health. It is never my intention to give a patient such a forbidding diet that he can't socialize. A diet should be designed to allow the patient to enter his ideal blood-type diet at his own pace, with enough flexibility so that he can eat out at a restaurant or a friend's house and still get the food he requires. I never recommend a diet that I myself could not live with. While a health regimen may curb a person's eating habits, it is not meant to be so severe that it creates tension or rigidity in his personality, thereby defeating its purpose. To illustrate my methods, I will outline how each blood type should eat on a daily basis as he slowly, gradually works into his recommended diet.

Beginning with a person who is a type A, the following would be my recommendations for a *general* regimen.

TYPE A

Upon rising, before breakfast, the A should drink a glass of lemon juice and water (half a squeezed lemon in a glass of lukewarm water) to help eliminate the mucus which developed overnight from his throat, chest and stomach. This also encourages a healthy bowel movement. After a half-hour to forty-five minutes, he can have a glass of grapefruit or diluted orange juice (half water, half juice to weaken the acidity level), or a fruit such as half a grapefruit or cantaloupe. After waiting another half-hour to prevent the mixing of fruit or fruit juice with his breakfast (which would inhibit proper digestion), he can have eggs or cereal and bread.

As I have explained, dairy products such as eggs, milk and cheese are mucus-forming, and the inner kernel of the wheat grain is highly acid-forming to the A's body, therefore these foods should be slowly processed out of his diet in the first month of step two. Having reduced or eliminated fried foods in step one, the A should now eat his eggs boiled, poached, or coddled. He should also try to reduce the number he eats every day. Most egg-eaters have two a day but whatever his current consumption, he should try to bring it down to four or five eggs a week. If he's already at this level, he should try to reduce consumption to two or three a week.

Many people believe that eating the right foods is all there is to a proper diet, but that's only part of it: how foods are combined is equally important. Proteins such as eggs, and carbohydrates, like toast and cereal, should *never* be eaten at the same meal. On those mornings when the A does not eat eggs, he can have a cup of one of several types of cereals. Since he has now reduced or eliminated sugared or processed cereals, such as Rice Krispies, Corn Flakes or Sugar Smacks, he should now select his breakfast grains from oatmeal, soy/wheat, cornmeal or plain soy flakes (the latter are best for his body because of a high alkalinity level). A small amount of honey can be mixed with the cereal instead of white or brown sugar along with whole raw milk diluted with water, skim milk, skim milk diluted with water or (preferably) soy milk, a vegetable protein which is not mucus-forming in the body.

Now that he has reduced or eliminated white and enriched breads, the A may have a slice or two of whole-wheat bread with the cereal. Eventually, however, the A should try to switch to the more alkaline soy/wheat, soy/sunflower or sprouted wheat breads (sprouted breads are made entirely from sprouts and water and are not acid-forming in the A's body).

Liquids, including water, milk, tea or coffee, should not be drunk during the meal because they can retard enzymatic action in the stomach during digestion. If the A wants to drink a liquid, or must have his morning cup of coffee, it would be best if he waited a half-an-hour to forty-five minutes after breakfast in order to allow the initial stages of digestion to begin.

Lunch for the A should be a vegetarian meal. If this is not desirable, or can't be started right away, the A should slowly work his way off meat lunches. Cold cuts, hamburgers, frankfurters and pizza were reduced or eliminated in step one and now he should substitute such easily digested animal proteins as broiled chicken or baked flounder. Gradually instead of these foods he should begin having a medium-sized salad consisting of, for example, lettuce, cucumbers, celery, alfalfa or mung-bean sprouts and grated raw zucchini for lunch. Tofu should also be included in this meal to provide his protein (a square of tofu is as high in protein as a quarter of a chicken).

Whole-wheat or soy bread may be eaten with a pat of unsalted butter or soy or safflower margarine. If dairy products are desired, he may have a small helping of ricotta or cottage cheese, or a cup of yogurt. However, cheese and bread should not be mixed at the same meal. Liquids should again not be drunk with the meal.

After a half-hour to forty-five minutes, the A may have fruit such as a grapefruit, peach or strawberries. If he has an occasional urge to backslide and eat an animal-protein meal of chicken or fish, this is perfectly okay: he should not be unreasonable in his discipline.

Dinner, like lunch, should eventually be a vegetarian meal. It is common, however, in most American families to eat meat seven nights a week, and it may take some doing to break this habit! If beef and pork have reduced or eliminated in step one, the A's dinner should not consist of chicken or turkey or fish. If beef and pork products have not been completely eliminated from his diet, he should try to restrict them to one or two nights a week.

After about a month, the A should introduce a vegetarian dinner consisting of a mixed green salad, steamed vegetables and a grain, such as brown rice, one night a week. When he feels that the vegetarian night has become an accepted part of his diet, he should allow another night for a vegetarian menu, perhaps substituting for brown rice another grain such as millet, buckwheat or wheat pilaf. As each additional vegetarian dinner is introduced, the A should try to eliminate the meat proteins from his diet: first beef and pork if he is still eating them, then chicken or turkey, and finally fish. This should be attempted over a three- to five-month period, giving the body the time to adjust to the taste and nutrients of vegetables and grains.

Here again, as with lunch, if there is a need to have a meat meal, such as chicken or fish, I suggest that the A do so without feeling guilty; getting emotional or "uptight" will only create tension and toxicity in his body. However, the A should remember that all meats are acidic-forming and mucus-forming in his body, and if continued for an extended period of time, can contribute to the gradual development of such diseases as arthritis, heart disease or rheumatism. A story I usually tell my patients, regardless of their blood type, takes place during World War II, when the Germans occupied France and Norway. The German soldiers, who had confiscated butter, eggs, thick cream and cheeses from the farmers, incurred an increase in cardiovascular-related diseases, while the incidence of heart disorders and arthritis decreased proportionately among the conquered! A recent study of the world's youth by the American Health Foundation has shown that children in countries such as Finland, who consumed large quantities of cheese, butter and eggs, had inordinately high cholesterol levels. In contrast, in Nigeria, where these foods are not eaten in such quantity, the children had a very low cholesterol level and the adult coronary disease rate was found to be minimal.

As he is changing his diet, the A should also begin to evaluate his exercise program. If it is a vigorous daily regimen, including jogging several miles a day or doing two hours of gymnastics, I suggest that he reduce his exercises. The A should not strain or excite his body, but seek to calm his nervous system: the best discipline for him would be Hatha Yoga. (Today, there are many good yoga teachers all across the country; in many states, yoga lessons are even given on television.) Beginning slowly, with five or six asanas (positions) the first week, he should gradually increase the number to about sixteen asanas, the full cycle for the intermediate student. As his kinetic energy is relaxed more of his real personality will emerge.

TYPE O

A regimen for a person with type-O blood is designed according to his need for protein. To sustain his strength, animal protein will be necessary five to seven times a week depending upon his occupation, physical regimen and general expenditure of energy. A vigorous physical-exercise program is fundamental to the O's well-being, and a daily program of an hour or two of exercise should be his goal (if he is of an appropriate age and state of current health).

The daily diet for the O in step two would be as follows:

For breakfast, he can begin with a juice: orange, grapefruit, papaya or apple. Fresh-squeezed orange or grapefruit is preferable; if the juice is purchased in a bottle or carton, the O should make sure it is sugar-free. After waiting a half-hour to forty-five minutes, he can choose either a dairy or grain breakfast. Fried or scrambled eggs were reduced or eliminated in step 1, so the O will eat his eggs soft-boiled, poached or coddled. His rate of consumption should now be reduced to about six a week, and eventually to four or five a week, even though eggs are a high source of protein. With his eggs, the O can have a square of tofu or some soft cheese such as ricotta, cottage or farmer's cheese (unsalted cheese is preferable; hard cheeses such as cheddar or Jarlsberg should be avoided as they are usually prepared with a lot of salt and chemical preservatives.) If the O desires a glass of milk, he can have a half a glass of raw milk or a full glass of soy milk thirty to forty minutes after the meal.

On mornings when eggs are not eaten, the O may choose his

cereals from a wide variety such as bran, millet, wheatgerm, shredded wheat, rice, cornmeal, oatmeal, soy/wheat or virtually any wheat-derived grain, since these are far less acidic to the O than the A. If the O selects a mixed cereal such as granola or Familia, he should read the label carefully, for such cereals often combine dried fruit and brown sugar with the grains. These cereals should be strictly avoided because fruits and grains do not combine well. A rule of thumb to be remembered: just because a health food store carries a product does not necessarily mean it is good for *your* body . . . be discriminating.

With his cereal, the O can use raw milk, diluted raw milk, skim milk or soy milk and a small amount of honey. His selection of breads may include whole wheat, seven or ten grain, buckwheat loaf, Scandinavian crispbreads, or any of the soy loafs.

Lunch should be vegetarian for the O. Even the O, who requires a high-protein diet, should not eat meat more than once a day! Excessive meat and fat create toxicity. All meats—cold cuts, chicken, fish, veal and lamb—should be eliminated from his lunch even if the O has a demanding occupation or is very physically active. Sufficient protein will be provided through the dinner meal. However, if the O prefers to eat his main meal of the day at lunch, this would be okay, and I often recommend it. Meats can take up to three or four hours to be digested, and people often go to sleep with a full stomach, especially socially active people who don't dine until nine or ten o'clock at night. Eating meat in the middle of the day allows the body a longer time to digest these heavy foods.

If the O does eat his main meal in the evening, he should gradually reduce his intake of heavy meats from lunch. His best lunch would be a salad of lettuce, rugola, cucumber, squash, tomatoes, raddish, carrots and celery, and a square of tofu and/or a soft cheese for additional protein. If bread is eaten, cheese should be excluded.

An apple, orange or a bowl of blueberries can be eaten a half-hour to forty-five minutes later. If a beverage is desired, he should wait the same amount of time in order to prevent the retardation of the digestive process.

For dinner, the O who has reduced or eliminated pork and beef in step one, may have veal, lamb, turkey, chicken or fish as frequently as he wants. The more demanding his job or exercise program, the more that higher grades of protein, such as veal and lamb should be eaten. If he can get organic beef, calf's liver, kidneys, lung or heart, these make excellent sources of protein for him.

Animal proteins can be divided between higher and lower grade proteins. A suggested weekly diet for the O is to eat high-protein veal, lamb or kidney once a week, and select from low-protein chicken, turkey or fish the rest of the time. An O who has an office job, or who doesn't get out and exercise enough should reduce his intake of veal and lamb to once every two weeks; lower grade proteins such as chicken and fish should make up most of his protein intake. He may also, depending on his physical condition, want to include a vegetarian meal once or twice a week (brown rice, millet, barley or buckwheat, or a baked potato with a square of tofu to provide his protein requirement).

TYPE B

Before designing a diet for the type-B patient, I first have to determine the nature of his disorder. If an inventory of his physical condition reveals that his past and/or current illnesses are related to catarrh or mucus (asthma or arthritis for instance), I will have to put him on a modified non-mucus-forming diet similar to the A regimen. If he doesn't suffer from catarrhal-related ailments, but is fatigued and slightly depressed, I will recommend a type-O diet.

A "B" with a catarrhal nature has to greatly reduce his intake of dairy products, including butter, milk, cheese, eggs and yogurt. His typical breakfast begins with diluted grapefruit, orange or papaya juice. After waiting a half-hour or so, the B may have one or two soft-boiled or poached eggs. He should, however, have only about four eggs a week initially, and slowly reduce eggs to one or two a week. Unlike the A's regimen, this diet is only a temporary measure to hasten the elimination of mucus. The B will eventually be able to have three or four eggs a week.

If he prefers cereal for breakfast, I recommend that he make his selection from millet, soy/wheat, oatmeal or cornmeal. A spoonful of wheatgerm or bran may be added to his cereal once a week. Small amounts of honey may also be added, but all animal-derived milks should be *strictly avoided*. Alkaline-forming soy milk is best for the B but if animal's milk has to be used, he should choose raw milk diluted with water, skim, or diluted skim milk.

Since he is not limited in his diet only to soy products, the B has a wide selection of breads to choose from, including whole wheat, seven or ten grain, Scandinavian crispbreads, sprouted wheat or any of the soy loafs. However, as the key to the B's regimen is moderation, whole-wheat products (although not so acidic to the B as they are to the A) should be eaten only a few times a week, alternating with soy bread.

The B, like the other blood groups, may have a grapefruit, orange or strawberries after waiting the required time, or a beverage such as an herbal tea, or a cup of black coffee if he has not yet eliminated coffee.

For lunch, the B should, like the A and O, gradually work his way to a vegetarian selection. A mixed green salad, including celery, carrots, cucumber, squash and sprouts with a square of tofu for protein, plus a slice or two of bread would be a good typical lunch. Cheeses and yogurt should be strictly avoided during this cleansing period.

At dinner, the B should eliminate his intake of beef and pork and eat veal and lamb once a week, and chicken and fish once or twice a week. Lamb should then be reduced to once every two weeks, and chicken and fish increased to four times a week (two days of each). Eventually, the B should try to eliminate veal and lamb temporarily because it is acidic and mucus-forming within his body, and eat chicken and fish three nights a week, and a vegetarian dinner (salad, steamed vegetables and a grain such as brown rice, buckwheat or millet, or a baked potato) the other four nights.

As the B's condition improves and the concentration of mucus is eliminated from his body, he can slowly reintroduce dairy products and eat three to four eggs a week, and raw milk, soft cheeses and unsalted butter four times a week. Veal or lamb may again be eaten once a week.

If the B is not catarrhal in nature, I would suggest that he follow an adaptation of the O regimen. Breakfast, then, could include orange, grapefruit or papaya juice, an egg three or four times a week, tofu and cottage or ricotta cheese. Or he may substitute cereal, honey and milk and bread. Lunch should be vegetarian, with whole-wheat or soy bread and tofu, or tofu and a soft cheese with his salad. Dinner should be a selection of either veal, chicken, turkey or fish four or five times a week, and vegetarian meals on the remaining nights.

With the appropriate diet regimen, I recommend that the B follow a moderate physical-exercise program. Such exercises as jogging, hiking, swimming, bicycling, Hatha Yoga or T'ai Chi Ch'uan may be done on a daily basis, with the intensity of the program based on the patient's age and physical condition.

TYPE AB

The AB, who is virtually identical with the A, would in most cases be given a similar vegetarian regimen with the addition of fish one or two nights a week.

Like the A, the AB should begin his day by drinking a glass of lemon juice and lukewarm water to cleanse the mucus that has accumulated overnight in his stomach and throat. After waiting for about half an hour, the AB can have diluted orange, grapefruit or papaya juice, or half a grapefruit or cantaloupe. After another half-hour, the AB can have eggs (soft-boiled, poached or coddled), or a cereal such as oatmeal, cornmeal, millet, soy/wheat or soy flakes. A dab of honey, a small pat of butter or margarine, and diluted milk, skim milk or soy milk may be added to his cereal.

If he has eliminated white and enriched breads from his diet, the AB can now have whole-wheat bread, or preferably soy/wheat, soy/sunflower or sprouted-wheat bread with his cereal.

Any beverages may be drunk a half-hour to forty-five minutes after the meal.

For lunch, the AB should first reduce his meat intake, gradually cutting out cold cuts, hamburgers, frankfurters, and substitute chicken and fish, introducing a vegetarian lunch menu after about a month. Each week he should include another vegetarian meal (with a square of tofu) in his diet. Cheeses and yogurt should be limited to once or twice a week and eventually be completely eliminated.

Fruit such as a peach or papaya may be eaten, or a beverage drunk, about three-quarters of an hour after lunch.

The elimination of meat at the dinner meal should be a step-by-step process for the AB. Once beef and pork have been eliminated, dinners may include veal, lamb, chicken or fish. Veal and lamb and then chicken should gradually be eliminated from his diet. Fish meals should be reduced to three or four a week and vegetarian dinners introduced. The balance the AB is seeking is five or six nights of vegetarian dinners, consisting of a salad, steamed vegetables, a potato, or a grain such as brown rice, barley or cornmeal, or a spinach or Jerusalem artichoke pasta, and fish on the remaining nights.

During step two, the AB should examine his current physical-exercise program. A vigorous regimen should be reduced because the AB, like the A, has a sensitive constitution that must be soothed and calmed. Jogging several miles every day or working out in the gym an hour or two is too demanding for his highly strung system. Hatha Yoga, T'ai Chi Ch'uan or light jogging or

84

swimming several times a week is the discipline I suggest for him. His true nature and greatest feeling of well-being will be attained when his body is relaxed.

Once the patient has eliminated the processed and refined foods in step one, and has settled into the general regimen for his blood type, he can, if he elects, go further into healing his specific condition. Step three, the third and final phase of the diet can be worked into at different times of the patient's regimen. Just when the patient embarks upon step three depends upon his desire to heal himself, or upon the severity of his illness. In some cases, the diet I recommend may be more stringent than the general diet for his blood type, or even temporarily contradict the ideal diet to hasten the purification of the body.

Often before advancing into the more specific diet, a patient experiences an overall reduction of symptoms and a revitalized feeling of well-being. This is an indication that his body is undergoing the healing process owing to his adherence to the recommended diet. There are numerous case histories in my file of people who healed dramatically, unexpectedly just by staying on their regimens. A woman in her forties who is an AB type described herself as "suffering for years with such severe back troubles and aches and pains in my neck and elbows that I've had to sleep on top of a hard board and run an electric moist air heating pad up and down my body for an hour before getting out of bed," found that after only two months on her modified vegetarian regimen, "the backaches and stiffness in my neck have disappeared and I no longer wake up in the morning wondering if I'll be able to get out of bed and move."

A man who had temporarily lost his hearing in his left ear, but who actually came to me seeking help for his crippling case of sciatica, was greatly surprised that the non-mucus-forming diet I recommended (he was type A), not only relieved him of the agonizing pains in his back and leg, "but as a bonus, my left ear cleared up, and I can hear normally again." A teenage girl who had tried to be a vegetarian but whose type-O body required a high-protein diet, came to me disheartened because her once long and beautiful fingernails were now constantly breaking and brittle. Two weeks after she had gone on a high animal-protein diet she sent me a jubilant postcard, "I just observed my first change: my fingernails are growing again and they are stronger . . . who knows what else will happen!"

Like the results seen at step one, these responses can also be a "false high." A person will recover his strength and health, and often feel tremendous surges of energy. He'll suddenly become the life of the party, or will undertake new hobbies and projects. However, not until the underlying causes of his disorders are taken care of by reducing toxicity levels, repairing damaged tissues, and soothing inflamed body organs, will his energy level peak. His body can still be vulnerable to illness if he simply remains at this step of the diet or if he begins to backslide and eat undesirable foods. The direction of his diet, even when his health is fully recovered, must always be toward simpler, more harmonious foods.

As there are many causes of illness, determining the specific cause of the disorder is fundamental in providing a total cure. In designing a diet for an A with arthritis, for example, I believe that it is of paramount importance that the patient eliminate high-fat dairy products and animal proteins, which form mucus and are acidic within his body. In doing so, the A reduces the catarrh and uric acid, which he has difficulty eliminating and which lodge in his joints to cause aches and swelling. The reduction of fat intake also helps to prevent further clogging of his arterial vessels, which may obstruct the normal flow of blood to his heart and other areas of his body. So, for the arthritic A, I have found that these disorders can be corrected when he has worked his way into step two.

However, in the case of an O who requires a high animal-protein diet, and who is suffering with arthritis or a heart condition, step two would not completely remedy the cause of his problems. In fact, if he continued to follow this diet it could worsen his illness.

Let's see why. As we've seen, consuming animal protein three times a day is excessive, even for the O's high-vibrational body. Forty percent of a person's fat intake is derived from animal protein and dairy products. Eating meat, cheese, eggs and yogurt in abundance places an enormous strain on the digestive and circulatory systems and deposits a dangerous amount of acids and fat into the bloodstream.

Once the O has successfully adapted to step two, by eliminating beef and pork and eating the variety of meats I have suggested, I recommend that he lean toward the A regimen. Meat meals should be cut from five to seven times a week to three or four (depending on the degree of his illness). In addition, he should reduce his egg intake to two a week, and temporarily eliminate other dairy products such as milk, cheese, butter and yogurt.

If the person is suffering with arthritis, he should try to eat fish, which is leaner than veal, lamb or chicken, and soy products, such as tofu, and soy margarine instead of cheese and butter made from whole milk.

The O with a coronary condition can eat both fish and chicken and should substitute soy products for animal-derived foods when possible. Depending upon the severity of his disorder, he may be able to eat yogurt and cheese (preferably made from goats' milk) once or twice a week.

When his condition improves, I will again examine his iris. If I observe a shortening of the line over the corresponding position for the adrenal glands, which denotes a lessening of arthritic aches and swellings, or of the line over the heart and circulatory areas, which suggest a reduction of vascular pressure and deposits, I will change the diet. Now, the O may gradually increase his intake of dairy products and reintroduce such meats as veal, lamb and chicken into his diet.

A "B" suffering with similar ailments must lean toward the A regimen if an accumulation of catarrh exists. If he is experiencing arthritic aches and swellings, he should suspend his intake of eggs, cheese, butter and milk. Since he does not need daily animal protein, the B should temporarily refrain from eating veal, lamb, and chicken, and eat fish three times a week to prevent an increase of mucus, acids and fat in his system. During this time he should eat tofu four or five times a day, eat soy flakes and soy granules rather than oatmeal or millet and increase his intake of soy beans to twice a week.

If his condition is a coronary disorder or a circulatory illness, the B should have fish twice a week and chicken once. Dairy products should be avoided. (If this is objectionable to the patient, I usually suggest that he have yogurt and cheese made from goats' milk once a week.) Tofu should be eaten four or five times a day to fortify his strength and promote tissue repair.

An AB with these ailments should follow a non-mucus-forming vegetarian diet similar to the A's regimen. Depending upon his energy requirements, however, he may include fish once a week.

When I treat a disorder such as high blood pressure, there are certain changes in step three that I make for all blood types. Because the blood vessels have become lined with fatty deposits that cause a loss of elasticity, they are no longer responding properly to the pulsations of the heart. This creates an increase in blood pressure. A common method of reducing high blood pressure is to eliminate the fatty deposits from the circulatory system and consequently reduce the strain on the heart. This, in my opinion, is only half a treatment.

Eating meats, dairy, fat, and fried and sautéed foods has been associated with the accumulation of arterial deposits. Therefore, these foods should be refrained from or reduced (according to the person's blood type) when such a condition exists. However, often overlooked in the treatment of high blood pressure is the effect of impaired kidneys on the cardio-vascular system.

The kidneys are organs of elimination, and when they are damaged, cannot efficiently filter impurities from the blood. I have found that this allows mucus and fat to circulate and line the arterial walls. Therefore, it is necessary to flush the morbid matter congesting the kidneys out of the body. A patient with high blood pressure should drink ten to twelve glasses of water a day to help eliminate waste. Many people think that any liquid will serve the same purpose, but I have discovered that such fluids as coffee, tea or juice are more viscous than water and will not effectively filter impurities from the kidneys.

Dandelion tea, which purifies and helps heal kidney tissue, should also be drunk four or five times a day, and asparagus, in my experience one of the best healers of the kidneys, should be eaten as often as possible. Spices, including such herbs as tarragon, basil, oregano, chives and rosemary, should be temporarily eliminated because they can irritate impaired kidney tissue and worsen the condition.

People of all blood types should also eat the inner rind of citrus fruits (the O and B from the grapefruit or orange; the A and AB from the grapefruit only). The rind (the fleshy white layer separating the skin from the juicy pulp) has a high concentration of rutin, a nutrient which increases the permeability and strength of the capillaries. I believe that rutin is beneficial to patients with high blood pressure.

Lastly, salt should be removed from the diet of all patients with cardiovascular disease. Although normally the O and B can eat sea salt in moderation, they too must temporarily suspend its consumption if they have high blood pressure. Salt causes retention of water in the body, resulting in an increased amount of pressure on the blood vessels. Salt in all forms should be avoided, for example butter should be sweet instead of lightly salted, and only unsalted seeds should be eaten.

The results from step three of the diet can be remarkable, even profound. These letters from people who have undergone the full healing program will show you the powers of the Nature Cure.

When I came to you, I had a gallstone. I had been told that there was no alternative to an operation. I also had high blood pressure and swollen ankles. My improvement during the year that I've been on my diet has been extraordinary. At 50, I feel better than I did at 20. The gallstone, as you know, has dissolved, and I no longer am bothered with those abrupt sharp pains in my kidney. My blood pressure is normal and my ankles hardly ever swell anymore. My figure is beautifully slim, a "side effect" achieved with no effort at all, other than eating substantial healthful meals. Everyone comments on the clarity of my complexion and I always have boundless energy.

A young man in his midtwenties wrote:

When I came to you for treatment, I had excruciating abdominal pains, bad digestion, constant constipation, constant nasal congestion and bleeding from the rectum. It's been like this for me since I was four. The diet of fruits and vegetables, which I thought was a joke, saved me. It is a miracle that I no longer am in constant pain. I don't like to throw the word "miracle" around freely; but in my case, after suffering with these ailments for over twenty years, virtually my entire life, it is the only word that seems appropriate.

This next letter is from a woman suffering with one of the oddest complications I have ever come across.

Not being able to breathe properly *outside* the city limits, in fresh, clean air, would seem an unbelievable complaint. But there it is: I used to choke and get spasmodiclike heavings. I also almost always suffered with great discomfort in warm weather and had eczema on my elbows and hands. Nevertheless, you found the diet that was perfect for me. I admit I had to learn to like okra and tofu. Soy beans were also not one of my favorites, and I missed spinach quiche, cheddar cheese and vanilla ice cream. But after five months on the diet I can breathe! I am not congested and I no longer get those spasmodic attacks. I recently took a pleasant trip to the Bahamas and felt no discomfort from the heat or sun. As for my eczema, that's going to take a little longer. But, it's already reduced to the size of a dime on my right hand. All this without allergy tests, needles, and drugs.

I have found that during the final stages of the diet, many deep-healing processes are simultaneously activated. They are not always predictable or completely understood. One such peculiar happening is that often during the healing process, years of accumulated wastes, and actual illnesses that were in the past suppressed by drugs, reemerge. One teenage girl that I treated for psoriasis is a good example of this. Like many of my patients, she sought me out after many unfruitful experiences with conventional medicine. During the treatments, she made marvelous progress in cleansing her body and healing her sores. But, her body healed itself in an odd pattern: taking three steps forward and two steps back! Most of the sores would heal and then some would return. Eventually her skin became smooth and supple, but the odd fluctuations of the healing process often disturbed the girl for she couldn't understand that the recurrence of her condition, for a period of time, was part of the cure.

Nature is unpredictable and mysterious in the way She heals. However, a patient can always be assured that there will be a cure, a truthful cure, from "within the body out."

Nature works slowly. This can't be emphasized enough: the return of health rests totally on the patient's perseverance in following a recommended diet. Only his desire for health will bring health; only his willingness to alter past habits will implement it.

6

How Do *You* Feel?

In the last chapter, I described how I create a Natural health care program. One of the myths about Natural Healing in this country is that anybody can read a book about it, eat "Natural foods," and take vitamins and herbs, thereby healing an illness; this is like suggesting that a person could cut his own body open and perform major surgery on himself. However, I do feel that there are active measures you can take to nourish your body and help correct some of your discomforts.

Before outlining the steps you will follow in order to design your personalized diet program, I want to address those people already involved in a nutritional regimen such as macrobiotics, vegetarianism or raw foods.

Many people who come to me already follow a health regimen, but want additional advice on, for instance, vitamins and herbs. These people claim they feel wonderful, that their present diet has made all the difference in their lives, and that they don't really need a customized program for their body. My response to these people, and to any readers who feel the same way, is this.

The elimination of highly acidic foods, rich sauces and gravies, heavy meats, buttery pastries, and foods containing artificial coloring, preservatives and chemical additives, immediately reduces the stress put on all the body's systems. A body no longer ingesting greasy, heavy foods and chemical compounds will suddenly be as spunky and light as a tugboat set free after pulling an ocean liner into port. Digesting these harmful substances has a phenomenally exhausting effect on the body.

Secondly, if you are currently following a regimen such as macrobiotics or vegetarianism, your body is being supplied with the essential basic nutrients found in fresh fruits and vegetables and grains, nutrients which are absent from commercially processed foods. In addition, the large amounts of roughage in fresh foods also helps to "sweep the body clean" of many lingering toxic wastes.

I often hear people on a vegetarian diet say that they don't feel as dense or bloated as they had when they ate meat and dairy products, and that their minds have never been clearer and more alert. However, and there should be no mistake about this, it is the elimination of vitaminless junk foods and the change-over to fresh fruits and vegetables that is responsible for flushing out undesirable toxins, nourishing the body with better grade nutrients and the consequent feeling of well-being.

Compared to the way the person felt before, any slight alteration in his diet will promote this type of physical euphoria, but it is a trap which I have called a false high.

No single regimen is right for all people. Although your body may recover a degree of health while on a vegetarian or macrobiotic diet, or your blood pressure may be reduced by cutting out certain foods, these practices are like fool's gold. In the long run they can be detrimental to your health because they do not take into account your individual constitution and nutritional requirements. I have seen it happen time and time again.

One case that particularly stands out in my mind is that of a middle-aged man who had emphysema. A type B, he required a combination animal-protein/vegetable diet. But, after reading several health books and consulting a supposedly knowledgeable friend, he thought he could cure himself. He put himself on a

94

completely vegetarian diet, eating a fruit bowl for breakfast, vegetable soup for lunch, and a large mixed salad with one slice of whole-wheat bread for dinner. His only sources of protein were from almonds and alfalfa sprouts.

Such diets have been successful in cleansing the body by helping to rid it of mucus and irritants in the respiratory system. However, I warned him that the lack of protein would eventually catch up with him, weaken his body and make it susceptible to other illnesses. During the six months he adhered to his diet, his body became so frail that a slight head cold developed into an advanced case of pneumonia. The man was rushed to the hospital half dead, placed in intensive care and immediately put on a high-protein diet. His medical doctor told him he had nearly starved himself to death. The man survived, and even though he made significant progress in controlling his emphysema, the complication that had ensued could have been avoided had he remained on a balanced diet according to his blood type.

So for you people who are already following a diet, I agree that it may seem successful and bring you a renewed feeling of vitality—but this is a short-term reaction. Over a long period of time, *a diet not suited to your specific constitution can be potentially harmful to your health.*

Before determining what diet is best suited for your needs, an analysis of your current state of health must be made. Your nutritional program will be based on the symptoms you are now experiencing and on your blood type. As I mentioned earlier, it is easy to find out your blood type: people who have been in the hospital, the armed services, who have given blood, women who have had children, have all been tested routinely for their type. If you don't know your blood type you can find it by tests performed by your family physician or at a local blood bank.

The following are some of the questions you should ask yourself in order to evaluate your present physical condition. Write your answers down. They will later help you to select your proper diet. Your notes will also serve as a reminder of your intentions and help you keep sight of your health goals.

1. Make a thorough analysis of your body's current state. Do you have any aches and pains? Do you have sinus or chest congestion? Do you get headaches? Stomachaches? Are you tense and nervous? Depressed? How would you rate your energy level: high or low? Do you have difficulty eliminating regularly?

Write down *all* your body discomforts.

2. After listing your symptoms, try to determine how often you have these discomforts and rate yourself as follows:

OCCASIONALLY:
Once or twice a week, lasting a few minutes in duration;
MODERATELY:
Every morning for ten or fifteen minutes;
CONSTANTLY:
Every day, the level of severity fluctuating throughout the day.

3. Now that you have determined the extent of your discomfort, think back and try to determine how long you have been suffering with these current problems. Also, try to remember any other similarly related illnesses or discomforts you may have had in the past. For instance, if you now suffer with a chest congestion, did you ever have other illnesses that affected the respiratory system, such as bronchitis or sinusitis?

4. Assess your concern for your discomfort. Are you depressed or made tense by it? Are you upset by it? Do you fear it? Be honest with yourself. Are you very upset? Or is it only a minor inconvenience? Do you find yourself preoccupied by it throughout the day? Is it affecting your work, family life, happiness? What do you think is causing your discomfort?

5. Decide how quickly you would like to help yourself. Think about how much health you would like returned to your body. Do you want to be completely healed? Or would you be satisfied if you were simply no longer made uncomfortable by your problem? How much are you willing to modify your present lifestyle to regain your health? As much as necessary? A little? How strict can you be with your diet? Can you avoid certain favorite foods? Or, will you always need to include them in your diet?

Can you give up drinking? Smoking? Are you really ready to start on a health program?

The rest of this chapter is devoted to helping you to create your individualized diet. You will see that I have prepared rating charts for each blood type. Each chart is divided into five levels to help you decide, based on your current state of health, which diet is right for you now. By referring to your evaluation of your present health, you will be able to slot yourself into the level that seems most appropriate to you and your condition.

If, for instance, you are just embarking on a nutritional program you may want to begin at level one, which is the general introduction to nutritional care. People already involved in a diet, or who are seriously ill and require more immediate care may choose to begin at a higher level. Those whose discomforts are moderate may want to begin at level three or four.

The ultimate goal for people who want to maximize their health and strength, is gradually to work toward the level (five) that is the ideal diet for your blood type. The diet, for example, of a type A who has reached his ideal diet (A–5 on the rating chart), is completely vegetarian, and free of whole-wheat products, almost all dairy foods, and fruits such as apples and pears.

In choosing the level at which you wish to begin, be sensible. Don't overextend yourself. Try not to be too ambitious or make drastic changes right away. It's good to turn over a new leaf and improve your eating habits, but not if it's going to upset you or your family. Move into a regimen slowly; eliminate your old eating habits one by one, replacing each with some of the ideas I suggest. If you enter a diet at a level you find too demanding, go back a step or two and start again at a lower level.

However, if you have a severe illness and need immediate care, I recommend that you begin at the highest level immediately and consult a qualified Natural healer or a sympathetic medical doctor. If you are in great pain or if your health is in a precarious state, do not try to do this program by yourself!

Indeed, it's probably a good idea before beginning these diets to seek professional guidance, regardless of your state of health. If you are under the care of a Naturopath, I advise you to consult him and explain the program you are about to follow. If you are not under the care of a Naturopath, or don't know where to find one, visit your family medical doctor. While he may not be in total accord with the Naturopathic approach to healing, he is certainly knowledgeable about the way the body works and will at least be able to guide you, and monitor your progress on the diet.

People with type-A or -AB blood should recognize that it may be difficult to adapt to a vegetarian regimen, therefore, they may want to work slowly into their program, taking perhaps eight months to a year to fully acclimate their bodies to the regimen. The O and B will find that they can make more rapid progress in adapting to their diets because the restrictions are not as extensive. In all cases, the stronger your will to ascend to your ideal diet, the greater the likelihood that health and vitality will be returned to your body.

Lastly, as I have explained, self-regulation and discretion are required in regard to the consumption of certain foods. If you are an O, for instance, and do not have a demanding occupation, or are not physically active, remember that you should reduce your protein intake. Similarly, if you are an A who is physically active, you may require fish or chicken several times a week to meet your demands.

Remember, in order to locate the proper level on your chart, you must refer to the symptoms you wrote down at the beginning of the chapter. If you are experiencing your condition occasionally (once or twice a week every couple of weeks) then your condition is probably not severe. You can begin your regimen at level number one. If you have a recurrence of your symptoms every day for about ten or fifteen minutes, your body requires more immediate attention and you should begin your program at level number three. For those of you whose symptoms are constant, persisting at various degrees of pain throughout the entire day, I recommend that you begin at level four or even five if possible, because your body is probably highly toxic and your organs may be badly inflamed or deteriorated.

Also, as a general rule, remember that the closer you move to the ideal of your blood group, the faster you will start to remedy some of your discomforts, for your body will be nourished with the vital nutrients it needs to promote tissue repair and revitalize your strength.

As I mentioned in the last chapter, certain disorders such as high blood pressure, arthritis or lung congestion, may necessitate an alteration of the diet common to your particular blood type. If you are an O who has consumed an excessive amount of meat, dairy and fat and now have a high-cholesterol count, or a heart disease, you should temporarily reduce your consumption of animal proteins, dairy products and eggs, even though O's ordinarily require a high-protein diet. If you are a B with similar disorders, you should tend toward the A regimen, instead of the O, and enter your program at the level appropriate to your condition. A's and AB's should follow their charts, also entering at a level based upon the severity of illness.

To help you make better use of the rating charts, the following are examples of the way I would assign a patient to his level, according to his blood type, age and illness.

When I treated a boy of eight who was a type B suffering with asthma, I started him on the modified A regimen, B3: catarrhal nature. Because an excessive consumption of dairy products is often the cause of this condition in children of his age, milk, cheese, eggs and yogurt were eliminated from his diet. As his asthma abated, I gradually changed his diet, working him up the chart to B5. Had the boy been older, fourteen or fifteen, I might have started him on a stricter diet, such as B4. However, strict and restrictive diets can be initially too demanding for a child. His emotional response might possibly undermine the effectiveness of the diet, and even worsen his condition.

I recommended A3 for a woman in her middle fifties who was suffering with gout and rheumatoid arthritis, with severely swollen wrists and ankles. Because I believe that conditions like this are often brought on by heavy meats in the diet and a regular intake of alcohol (and are especially common among people who lead an active social life), the diet I suggested was a strict vegetarian regimen. However, this woman found it too difficult to make this sudden change in her life-style, so I had to modify her regimen to one that was equivalent to A2. This slowed the healing process, yet nevertheless, within one month her swollen joints began to return to normal.

Before I diagnosed a woman in her twenties who was an AB suffering with a liver disorder, I first investigated her drug history. A sluggish liver, caused by the use of marijuana or hashish, is a phenomenon I have found in many patients who were in their late teens and early twenties in the 1960s. Toxicity levels are heightened in people who smoke pot and the result is damaged liver cells and body fatigue. This proved to be the case with this woman, so I recommended she stop smoking marijuana and begin her diet at AB3. I also advised her to be very patient during the treatments because in her condition, two or three years might be required to eliminate the toxicities and rehabilitate her liver.

A man, thirty years of age, who was an A suffering with acute sinusitis began his diet at A3. The elimination of dairy products and meats resulted in rapid improvements in his respiratory system. Congested mucus was broken up and eliminated, and the development of future congestion was prevented. The elimination of nasal sprays, antihistamines and other medications also allowed the mucus to be dispersed and discharged from his body.

A boy in his teens, who was an O with a recurrent case of acne, entered his diet at O3. However, I recommended that he reduce his consumption of meat and eat only fish, because meat has a higher uric acid and fat content and, in my experience, is often the main cause of skin eruptions. In addition, the boy drank ten to twelve glasses of water every day to purify his blood, and washed his face with a glycerine soap, which has a drying effect on pimples.

I strongly urged a man in his sixties, who was a type B suffering with a cardiac condition, to enter a highly restrictive diet because I believed that at his age, his arteries were so heavily clogged with fat and mucus he needed immediate deep-healing action. A disciplined man determined to regain his health, he began at B4: catarrhal nature. Within only two months, he had reversed many of the effects of years of bad eating, discharging an enormous amount of cholesterol while also strengthening his heart tissue and regenerating the flexibility of his arteries.

A woman in her middle fifties who was an O type experiencing extreme fatigue began her diet at O1, working her way to O4 over a period of one year. Her letter best described the progress she made. "During the past year I have been transformed from a vegetable to a healthy, functioning human being. Before seeing you, my situation was moving from bad to hopeless. I could remain out of bed for no more than an hour or two a day, in a state of fatigue and with great pain. I had been to many MDs, among them a well-known specialist. None of them had correctly diagnosed my illness or helped me. As I said, I now function as a normal healthy person. The diets you recommended for me, and which I followed to a 'T,' brought me back to life."

The diets I describe in these charts are only recommendations. They are also not entirely representative of a full Naturopathic treatment, which includes many therapies, some of which I mention in future chapters. However, these diets can be the beginning of your treatment as a unique individual.

7

How to Create
Your Own Diet

TYPE A

Level One

This is an evaluation step for those who are not yet following a dietary regimen, and are still eating commercially processed foods. The average American with type-A blood will have a long journey to level five, with many foods to eliminate from his diet as he makes the adjustment to a vegetarian life-style. The A will have to be patient in altering his diet, but it is not impossible, nor even terribly difficult. I, myself, am an A, and a product of a good Italian family—which means that I had my share of pasta, sausages and prosciutto to give up! Even though I had fond memories of spaghetti and clam sauce when I decided to change my eating habits, it only took about six weeks to reeducate my taste buds and embrace a new way of eating. Take it from me: your palate quickly loses its hunger for certain tastes; it's your thoughts you must master. Control your thoughts and in a short period of time you can switch from, for example, scungilli to a fresh mixed salad without feeling deprived.

Before you try to eliminate meat and dairy products from your diet, first substitute better quality equivalents for the foods you are now eating. Substitute whole grain breads and cereals such as whole wheat, rye, rolled oats and cornmeal for products made with white flour and chemical additives. Canned foods should be replaced by fresh fruits and vegetables. Foods that have been preserved, flavored or colored, or are chemically synthesized should be totally eliminated. Buy your own pure ingredients— bake your own cake, prepare your own pasta dinner or steam your own whole brown rice. Others have said it before, but there is no doubt about it: you are what you eat. So think about what you are putting into your body. Be aware when you are eating, that food is fuel and a poor grade fuel is going to clog and rob your human machine of its potential energy and efficiency. Try to control your cravings.

The same kind of discretion should apply when selecting meats. It is crucial to avoid all packed meats such as canned ham, frankfurters and frozen fish. These products are usually preserved with salt and chemicals such as sodium nitrite, which has been linked with cancer. When shopping in the supermarket, be sure you buy only grade-A meats, with no additives. Meat should be well-sealed: exposure to air reduces its nutritional value. If you are now buying a lot of red meats such as chopped beef, steaks or roasts, or pork products, think about switching to veal, lamb, chicken and turkey. The latter choices are leaner, have less uric acid and concentrations of steroids and antibiotics. Fish is also lean and is a purer food than meat or poultry.

Your main consideration in buying any food should be: is this substance in its purest, simplest state; as close as possible to the state in which the fruit fell from the tree, the vegetable grew from the earth or the meat came from the animal?

Other factors that affect health and should now be examined are the amount of alcohol you drink, the number of cigarettes you smoke per day, and your current exercise program. Hard alcohol, which robs the body of many nutrients and debilitates the liver, should be eliminated, and replaced by moderate quantities of red or white wine. Consider the harm cigarettes inflict on the entire body: they weaken the lungs, destroy Vitamin C, which can lower your resistance against disease, and have been proved to contain cancer-causing agents. If you really want to recover your health fully, try to cut down with the goal of eventually eliminating cigarette smoking.

Lastly, evaluate the amount of physical activity you are currently engaged in. Is your occupation demanding? Do you exercise? How much? Are you exerting yourself? Remember the A should try to find peace through exercise and should not be stressing himself by attempting to be a marathon runner or a Charles Atlas.

The A should remain at this step for one to two months.

Level Two

At this level you will be concerned with narrowing your selection of foods. Your choice of meats should now only include veal, lamb, chicken, turkey or fish. Beef and pork products should be completely eliminated. Whole-wheat products and wheat-derived grains that were introduced in level one should now be alternated with soy products. For instance, whole-wheat bread may be eaten three or four times a week, on the other days select a soy loaf. Soy beans, soy flakes or granules should be substituted for millet, cracked wheat or buckwheat. A square of tofu should be eaten with every meal, too.

Dairy products should also be cut back. Milk should be diluted with water, soft cheese substituted for hard cheese, eggs reduced to four or five a week, and yogurt eaten only twice a week. Soy milk may be substituted for raw milk. Goats' milk products are better than raw milk, cheeses and yogurt.

You should eat vegetables steamed, not raw, at this level. This will help the body adapt to these highly laxative foods, and have a gentler effect on the bowels than raw vegetables. As your body adjusts to fresh foods, which may happen at this level or later in the program, you can eat your vegetables either steamed or raw.

Lunch should gradually become a vegetarian meal. If you are not ready to have raw salads as your meal, make a plate of steamed vegetables. If your body adapts readily to raw foods, then prepare a salad to your liking, but omit your favorite salad dressing. From this point on, use only oil and lemon and a few herbs such as rosemary, oregano, basil or dill. Cider vinegar especially should be avoided as it is too acidic for your body. Sea salt should now be used instead of regular table salt. Kelp powder, which is beneficial to a hyperactive thyroid, may also be used as a condiment on salads, vegetables or meat dishes.

Stay on this diet for about two months.

Level Three

All animal protein except chicken and fish should now be eliminated from your diet. It is also recommended that you reduce your intake of animal protein and eat chicken and fish only twice a week. Your selection of fish should include: bluefish, salmon, cod, scrod, haddock, halibut, flounder, sole, red snapper, brook trout, sea trout and sea bass. Shellfish, such as lobster, shrimp and clams should be avoided, as should tunafish and swordfish.

Your other main meals of the week should be vegetarian. However, whole-wheat products should be eaten only once or twice a week, and grains should be limited to brown rice, barley, millet and buckwheat. Good substitutes for grains are sweet or white baked potatoes, acorn or butternut squash, or Jerusalem artichokes.

Dairy products should be substantially reduced. *All* milks—raw, skim or goats'—should be replaced by soy milk. Cottage, ricotta or farmer's cheese should now be eaten only once or twice a week. Eggs should be reduced to two a week.

Fruits and vegetables now begin to play a prominent role in your diet. Fruit should be eaten two to three times a day between meals, or you may make an entire meal of fruits, eating, for instance, a whole cantaloupe or a large bowl of blueberries. Apples and apple juice, however, should now be eliminated, as should oranges, orange juice, pears, mangoes and bananas. Such alkaline fruits as watermelon, papaya, grapefruit (an acidic fruit which has alkaline properties after digestion), honeydew and cantaloupe are preferable choices for the A. Tomatoes, avocados, spinach and cabbage should now be strictly eliminated from salads.

This diet should be followed for about three months.

Level Four

All meats should now be completely eliminated from your diet. However, if you have difficulty making this adjustment at this level, or if you are under physical stress and still require animal protein, eat fish two or three times a week. All lunches and dinners, barring these exceptions, should be vegetarian meals. All cheese and dairy products should now also be eliminated from your diet. Eggs should be reduced to one a week. Because the white of eggs is primarily albumin, which tends to create gas in the A, egg white should be cut away and only the yolk of the egg eaten.

All whole-wheat grains and wheat-derived products should now be eliminated. Only soy products should be eaten.

Pumpkin and sunflower seeds and almonds and brazil nuts should now become an integral part of your diet. Eat a handful of nuts or seeds a day as a source of protein. Sprouts from alfalfa, mung beans, lentils and aduki seeds should become an important part of your diet because they are rich in minerals and also have a high vegetable protein content. Lima, soy and kidney beans should be eaten for their protein. Eat a square of tofu four to five times a day.

Brown rice should be eaten only twice a week for it can be too acidic for the A.

Include a tablespoon of olive oil on your salads or steamed vegetables every day. It has a good nutrient value and aids in digestion and elimination.

This step should be worked into over a period of about four to five months.

Level Five

All meals should now be vegetarian. All grains and breads should be soy-derived. One egg may be eaten a week; all other dairy products should be eliminated from the diet. Brown rice may be eaten once or twice a week.

Seeds, sprouts and tofu should be eaten every day as the main sources of protein. Fruits and vegetables are now the major source of all other nutrients.

This is the ideal menu for the A, and the goal of your regimen. It should be worked into slowly, with great deliberation, and at your own pace.

TYPE O

Level One

Eliminate processed and refined foods. Substitute whole-wheat products for breads made of white or enriched flour and do not eat processed cereals. Introduce whole-grain cereals such as millet, oatmeal, cornmeal and soy flakes to replace sugared and puffed breakfast cereals.

Reduce beef and pork products. Select animal protein from veal, lamb, calf's liver, chicken, turkey, the internal organs of organically raised cattle (kidneys, heart, lungs) and fish. Eliminate commercially produced dairy products, and choose milk, cheese, yogurt and butter made from raw cows' milk or goats' milk.

Eliminate fried foods. Reduce alcohol consumption and cigarette smoking. Substitute honey for white or brown sugar.

Evaluate your physical exercise program. Your goal is to create a vigorous regimen appropriate to your age and physical condition. An hour or two of exercise such as jogging, swimming, bicycling or gymnastics every day will greatly benefit you now.

Work into this step over a period of a month to a month-and-a-half.

Level Two

Animal protein should be eaten once a day every day. Choose one from the recommended selection in level five. Soft cheeses, including ricotta, farmer's, cottage and mozzarella may be eaten five times a week. A half a glass of whole milk may be drunk every day; and you can also have six eggs a week, and yogurt twice weekly.

You may eat whole-wheat products as often as you like, and you can also choose from such cereals as millet, oatmeal, cornmeal, soya/wheat, shredded wheat, wheatgerm and bran.

If you are younger than thirty, you may use butter made from raw cream but in moderation. O's over thirty, (the age at which your body's systems begin to slow and become more susceptible to the buildup of fatty deposits in your circulatory system) should switch to margarines made of such polyunsaturated oils as safflower, sunflower or soy. Cold-pressed oils can be mixed with lemon or with apple-cider vinegar and your choice of herbs for salad dressing.

Sea salt may be used in moderation; but kelp powder should be used sparingly because its rich iodine content may overstimulate your thyroid gland and increase your metabolic rate.

Vegetarian lunches should be introduced into your diet once or twice a week.

This step can be adapted over a period of two months. Once you have reached this stage successfully, there will be little change in your diet as you work toward level five, the ideal diet.

Level Three

Refer to level two for your allowed intake of animal protein.

Whole milk should now be reduced to four glasses a week, alternating with either skim or soy milk. (Regardless of the amount of cows' milk you drink, you may drink several glasses of soy milk a day.) Soft cheeses mentioned in level two may be eaten four times a week, yogurt twice a week. You should now lower your intake of eggs from six to four a week.

Lunches should now be vegetarian four to five times a week.

Olive oil should now be introduced in your diet. Take a tablespoon every other day to assist digestion and promote elimination.

Your physical regimen should now be fully created; to stimulate your body, take cold showers, hip baths and saunas regularly.

Unless you are suffering with a serious illness, you can take three to four months to work into this program.

Level Four

Continue to follow the regimen outlined in level three with these changes: lunch (if it is not your main meal) should now be totally vegetarian; in addition, eat a square of tofu with every meal for additional protein.

Level Five

The ideal O diet is as follows: oatmeal, soya/wheat, cornmeal, millet, shredded wheat, wheatgerm or bran for breakfast with diluted skim milk or soy milk and a dab of honey. Bread may be selected from whole-wheat or soy loafs.

Lunch, or the meal other than the main meal, should be entirely vegetarian, consisting of mixed salads and sprouts, with seeds or almonds. Tofu should be eaten four times a week, and you may eat soft cheeses four times a week, and yogurt twice a week. Four eggs are your weekly allowance.

The main meal of the day should be meat. The best balance is veal once a week, lamb and calf's liver once every two weeks, chicken or turkey twice a week, internal organs (if available) once a week and fish the remaining nights. Remember you must adapt your protein intake to your individual condition.

TYPE B

Midway in characteristics between the A and O, the B has a tendency to react like an A with a catarrhal nature, or like an O in an unbalanced state of health. This condition I call Fatigued B. An inventory of your symptoms will reveal which way the regimen will be directed.

110

Level One

Regardless of your current physical tendencies, you should begin your program by eliminating processed and refined foods. Candies, soda pop, chocolate syrup, canned foods and convenience dinners should be reduced as much as possible. Sugar should be replaced by honey. Whole grains should be substituted for instant and processed cereals. Introduce millet, soya/wheat, cornmeal, whole oats or buckwheat into your diet. Whole-wheat products should be substituted for refined-flour products.

Beef and pork should be reduced as much as possible, substituting lamb, veal, chicken or turkey and fish. Eggs should be organic and cheeses should be made from raw goats' milk. Coffee and tea should be replaced by a coffee substitute such as Pero or Pioneer; and hard alcohol with red or white wine, preferably mixed half-and-half with charged water.

All fried and sautéed foods should now be eliminated. Meats and fish should always be eaten broiled or baked, eggs boiled or poached and vegetables steamed.

Your physical-exercise program should now also be examined. Your goal is a moderate program of activities such as jogging, swimming, hiking, bicycling, gymnastics, calisthenics or Hatha Yoga. If your exercise program has been strenuous, reduce it now.

This level should be followed for about a month.

Level Two

Animal protein, such as veal, lamb, chicken, turkey or fish should be eaten once every day. Whole-wheat products should be alternated with soy products. Soy bread, soy wheat cereal, soy flakes and granules should be eaten four times a week, whole-wheat products, three. Tofu squares should be eaten four times a week.

Lunch should be vegetarian three times a week. Apple cider vinegar can be used with a polyunsaturated oil (safflower, sunflower or soy) on salads twice a week; the other days lemon should be mixed in the dressing. Sea salt and kelp powder may be used in moderation as condiments.

Fruits should be eaten three times a day between meals. Alternate steamed and raw vegetables in order to allow the body to adapt to the laxative effect of raw vegetables.

You should now start reducing your dairy products. Soft cheeses such as ricotta, cottage or farmer's cheese can be eaten four times a week, yogurt two or three times a week and eggs should be cut back to five or six a week. If you use milk, drink raw cows' or goats' milk, but only four or five glasses a week. Start introducing soy milk as a milk substitute.

This diet should be followed for about two months.

Level Three

Depending upon whether the nature of your body is catarrhal (retaining a lot of mucus) or fatigued, you should follow one of these two diets.

CATARRHAL NATURE:

Veal and lamb should be completely eliminated from your diet. Eat chicken or turkey once a week and fish twice a week. Recommended fish include: cod, flounder, red snapper, bluefish, halibut, salmon, sea trout and sea bass. Shellfish should be avoided. Your other dinners should be vegetarian, for example, a salad, steamed vegetables, a sweet potato or a grain such as brown rice.

At this time do not eat whole-wheat products. Use soy products instead. Dairy foods should be greatly reduced and soy milk should replace raw cows' or goats' milk. You may eat soft cheeses only once or twice a week, and only two eggs a week. Tofu should be eaten four times a day.

Continue to eat fruit three times a day between meals. Apples and apple juice should be temporarily eliminated because of their high acidity level, and oranges, orange juice, bananas and mangoes should also be avoided. Alkaline-forming fruits such as grapefruits, cantaloupe and watermelon are better for you during this period. Lunches should be completely vegetarian.

Follow this diet for three to four months.

FATIGUED B:

Veal and lamb should be eaten once a week, chicken or turkey twice a week and fish the remaining nights. Soft cheeses can be eaten three times a week, yogurt twice a week. You may have four to five eggs a week. A glass of cows' or goats' milk may be drunk three or four times a week.

You need to increase your protein intake, therefore, eat a square of tofu five times a day; and have soy protein drinks before breakfast and dinner (soy protein powder is available at any health food store). Stir a tablespoon-and-a-half of powder into a glass of water to make the drink.

Whole-wheat products may be alternated with soy products (whole wheat three times a week, soy, four times a week). Brown rice may be eaten two or three times a week, and other grains such as buckwheat, millet or barley may also be eaten in place of brown rice. All lunches should now be vegetarian.

Olive oil should now be introduced in your diet to encourage proper digestion and healthy elimination. Take one tablespoon every other day.

Physical exercise should be reduced if your body is greatly fatigued; if not, an hour's exercise may be taken four times a week.

This regimen should be followed for three to four months, or until strength has been returned to your body.

Level Four

CATARRHAL NATURE:

As the concentration of mucus is broken up and eliminated from your body, certain foods that were reduced or eliminated in level three may now be gradually reintroduced. Veal may again be eaten once a week. Chicken and turkey should now be eaten once or twice a week, and fish twice a week. The other main meals should be vegetarian.

Whole-wheat products, such as bread or soy/wheat cereal, may be eaten once a week. Grains such as millet, barley or buckwheat should be reintroduced and eaten once a week. You may continue to eat brown rice once a week.

Soft cheeses may be eaten twice a week and yogurt once a week, and you may have three eggs a week. Two to three glasses of raw cows' or goats' milk per week may be reintroduced in your diet. Soy milk may be drunk as often as desired. You may now have apples and apple juice once a week. Oranges may also be eaten once a week. Lunches should be vegetarian.

Follow this diet for two to three months.

FATIGUED B:

As the fatigue abates and your body regains its strength you may have veal once a week and lamb once every two weeks. Chicken or turkey may be eaten once or twice a week, reduce your fish meals now to twice a week. All other dinners should be vegetarian.

You should now reduce your consumption of soft cheeses to twice a week, and yogurt to once a week. Whole milk should be diluted with water, and eventually be replaced by skim milk, skim milk diluted in water, and finally, soy milk. Four eggs may be eaten a week, and continue to eat tofu four or five times a day. The soy protein drinks can now be eliminated. However, if you experience brief periods of fatigue, reintroduce this supplement in your diet.

Stay on this diet for two months.

Level Five

At the ideal level, the B should eat chicken or turkey twice a week, fish twice a week, and vegetarian dinners three times a week. Every other week you may substitute calf's liver, lamb or

114

veal for fish or chicken. If your occupation is not demanding, the combination of vegetarian/meat meals can be meat or fish three nights and vegetarian four nights.

Soft cheeses may be eaten twice a week, and yogurt once a week. You may also eat three eggs a week and drink two or three glasses of whole milk a week.

Whole-wheat and soy products should be alternated: soy products four times a week, and whole-wheat products, three. You may have brown rice once or twice a week, and other grains such as millet, cornmeal, or barley once or twice weekly.

Apples and oranges can be eaten twice a week, but avoid bananas entirely.

Sea salt and kelp powder may be eaten as desired.

TYPE AB

Level One

At this initial level, you should begin by eliminating processed and refined foods and those with chemical preservatives, artificial flavorings and additives. Coffee, tea, candies, soda pop, syrups, canned and prepared instant foods should now be reduced or eliminated. Bleached or enriched white-flour products should be replaced by whole-wheat products. Beef and pork products should be reduced, gradually being replaced by veal, lamb, chicken, turkey and fish.

Eat only those dairy products made from raw cows' or goats' milk. Avoid commercially processed milk. Eggs should be fertile, and cold-pressed oils should be used instead of commercially refined oils.

Fried or sautéed foods should be eliminated. Meat and fish should be broiled or baked, vegetables steamed, and eggs soft-boiled or poached. Substitute red or white wine for hard alcohol, and reduce the amount of cigarettes you are smoking.

Evaluate your exercise program. Your goal, like the A, is a

calming regimen. My recommended program includes Hatha Yoga, T'ai Chi Ch'uan, light jogging, hiking, swimming or a gym workout.

Follow this diet for a month or two.

Level Two

Meats that may be eaten at this stage include veal, lamb, chicken, turkey or fish. If possible your main meals should consist mostly of chicken or turkey and fish, instead of the more acidic meats, veal and lamb.

Whole-wheat products should now be alternated with soy products; whole wheat three and soy bread four times a week. Oatmeal, soy flakes, and soy granules are preferable to millet, farina, ground rice or corn. Wheatgerm and bran should be limited to once or twice a week.

Eggs should be reduced to four a week. Whole milk should be diluted, eventually substituting first skim milk, then skim milk diluted with water and, eventually, soy milk. Soft cheeses may be eaten two or three times a week, and yogurt twice a week.

Vegetables should be eaten steamed because if you are not accustomed to the laxative effect of raw vegetables your body needs time to adjust. Vegetarian meals should now be introduced at lunch (if this is not your main meal) at least two or three times a week.

Sea salt and kelp may be alternated as condiments. Apple-cider vinegar should be eliminated. Use lemon juice instead with oil and herbs to dress vegetables or salads.

This diet should be followed for up to three months.

Level Three

Veal and lamb should now be completely eliminated from your diet. Eat chicken or turkey twice a week, and fish the other nights. Recommended fish include: cod, salmon, halibut, flounder, sole, red snapper, sea or brook trout or sea bass. Shellfish and tuna and swordfish should be strictly avoided. If possible, introduce a vegetarian night once or twice a week and start cutting back slowly on your consumption of meat or fish.

Dairy products should now be slowly reduced. Raw milk should be replaced by soy milk. Soft cheeses should be reduced to twice a week, and yogurt to once a week. Eggs should be reduced to two a week.

Whole-wheat products should now be entirely eliminated. Substitute soy products. Grains such as millet, buckwheat or barley should be reduced to once every two weeks. Brown rice may be eaten once or twice a week.

Fruits and vegetables should now begin to play a prominent part in your diet. Fruits should be eaten three or four times a day between meals. Apples and apple juice should be eliminated, as should oranges and orange juice, bananas and mangoes. Vegetarian lunches should be increased to five or six a week, and vegetables may now be eaten both steamed and raw. An important addition to salads at this point are sprouted seeds including alfalfa, mung beans, lentils and soy beans.

Take up to three months to work into this diet.

Level Four

Fish consumption should now be reduced to three times a week, and all other dinners should be vegetarian. All lunches should now also be vegetarian. Cheese and yogurt should be eliminated from your diet and butter replaced by soy, safflower or lecithin margarine. All bread should be made from soy flour. Brown rice may be eaten once a week. Oatmeal and occasionally cornmeal may be eaten for breakfast.

Eat pumpkin and sunflower seeds and almonds every day for protein. Sprouts, which have a high mineral and protein content, should be an integral part of your daily diet. Mix them into salads or combine them with steamed vegetables. Lima, kidney or soy beans should also be eaten for protein. One or two eggs may be eaten a week, but discard the white part, which is gas-forming to the AB.

Fruits and vegetables should comprise an ever-increasing part of your diet (in Europe it is not uncommon to have a plain salad for breakfast).

Follow this diet for about three months.

Level Five

The ideal AB is a vegetarian except for two meals a week that should include a variety of fish. All breads and grains should be soy derived, and dairy products must be strictly avoided. One or two eggs may be eaten a week. Eat seeds and almonds each day now. Sprouts, an important source of protein, should be eaten several times a day. You may have brown rice once a week, oatmeal every day, cornmeal twice a week and bran once a week.

If you have a physically demanding occupation, you may want to add more fish or (occasionally) chicken to your diet to meet your energy requirements. This ideal level should be worked into at your own pace.

Although, as I have explained, different foods affect different blood types in dissimilar fashions, every nutrient possesses healing qualities. I have listed various foods that I recommend, with their healing qualities that I, as a practicing Naturopath, have discovered. Some things, of course, are appropriate for certain blood types and not others. Check your diet in earlier chapters.

HEALTH VALUE OF FOODS

Name	*Health Value*
Almonds	Aid in relieving nausea, dyspepsia; helps urinary excretion.
Apples	Help relieve indigestion and nourish a sluggish liver. Good nutrient source for those with rheumatism and gout.

118

Apricots................... Relieve constipation and are helpful for weight-reducing

Asparagus .... Revitalizes impaired kidneys and urinary tract. Helps soothe nerves.

Bananas .... Check diarrhea and help in gaining weight.

Barley .... Helps in reducing fever and building good blood.

Beans .... Supply important nutrients for those with anemia.

Blackberries/Blueberries ...... Excellent sources of nutrients for patients with rheumatism, gout, kidney trouble, sore throat, dyspepsia and diarrhea. Also help in checking cramps.

Bran .... Relieves constipation; good for the blood, teeth and bones.

Brazil Nuts .... Help cure malnutrition; nourish teeth and bones.

Broccoli................... Helps relieve constipation and high blood pressure. Aids in strengthening weak digestive glands, and curing neuritis.

Brussels Sprouts............. A tonic food. Help purify the body of catarrh, acidity and fatty deposits in the arterial vessels.

Cabbage.................... Helps purify the blood. Helpful in diseases such as asthma, high blood pressure, rheumatism and gout.

Cauliflower .... Helps control high blood pressure.

Celery .... Aids in relieving headaches, neuralgia, sciatica, arthritis.

Cherries.................... Relieve cramps, indigestion and anemia. Also helpful in discharging catarrh.

Chives .... Stimulates the urinary system. Helpful to a poor appetite, low blood pressure and asthma.

Corn...................... Aids in relieving constipation and low vitality. Also has important nutrients for cases of emaciation.

Cottage Cheese .... A good protein source. Also helps cleanse the large intestines.

Cranberries .... Relieve dysentery, flatulence and diarrhea. Help to check fevers and anemia.

Cucumbers .... Help reduce a fever, high blood pressure, nervousness, obesity, pyorrhea, skin eruptions, acidosis. A mild diuretic.

Currants .... A good nutrient source for patients with anemia, sore throat, asthma, coughs, bronchitis, weak heart, low blood pressure; also relieve constipation.

Eggplant .... Relieves colitis and stomach ulcers.

Eggs...................... Excellent protein source. Bone and muscle builders.

Elderberries................ Good for coughs, colds and sore throats.

Endive .... Nourishes the liver and heart.

Figs....................... A natural laxative; also help equalize blood pressure.

Flour (whole-wheat) .... Provides many minerals and

vitamins; helps build muscles, and promotes regular bowel movements.

Garlic...................... Good all-around stimulant. Aids in high and low blood pressure; also an antibiotic, helpful in curing colds, coughs, bronchitis.

Grapefruit .... Helps reduce fever; splendid for weight-reducing.

Grapes .... Enrich the blood. Act favorably in relieving dyspepsia, fevers, gout and rheumatism.

Honey .... Used in moderation, an all-around good food. Aids in digestion and improves blood circulation. Excellent for throat infections. Very effective in relieving constipation, asthma, and mucus accumulations.

Kale .... Helps improve problem skin; nourishes teeth and bladder.

Kelp....................... Helps normalize gland and cell action. Soothing to nervous disorders and anemic conditions. Strengthens thyroid gland.

Leeks .... Relieve coughs, colds and insomnia.

Lemons .... Nature's antiseptic. Reduces fever, purifies the blood and liver. An aid in nausea and obesity.

Lentils .... Help heal ulcerations of the digestive tract, and improve low blood pressure.

Lettuce.....................Helps relieve anemic conditions, insomnia and nervousness.

Mangoes ....Aid in kidney disorders such as nephritis; also help reduce fevers and acidosis.

Oats......................A body-builder. Good for hair, nails, teeth, glands and muscles.

Okra......................Soothing to stomach ulcers, sore throats. Helpful in relieving colitis and pleurisy.

Olive Oil..................Very nutritious, helps in gaining weight. Very effective for constipation.

Olives ....Good for anemia, nervousness, constipation and in gaining weight.

Onions....................Blood purifier; especially fine for insomnia, coughs and colds.

Oranges...................Excellent for reducing fevers. A general tonic for the blood and nerves.

Parsley....................Aids digestion. Strengthens prostate gland.

Parsnips...................Good for dyspepsia and diseases of the blood.

Peaches ....Blood purifier.

Pears......................Good laxative.

Peas (all varieties)...........Very nourishing, and muscle-building. Valuable in healing anemia and low blood pressure.

Pineapple..................Aids in weight-reducing, intestinal ailments and indigestion.

122

Plums. . . . . Stimulate the liver and help move the bowels.

Potatoes. . . . . Help in gaining weight; relieve diarrhea.

Prunes . . . . Nature's best laxative.

Radishes. . . . . Excellent in treating nervousness.

Raisins . . . . Blood purifier; also have a high iron content and help control anemia.

Raspberries . . . . Aid in alleviating cramps; also good for sore throats and fevers.

Rice (brown). . . . . Highly nutritious; helps strengthen all the body's organs. Also checks diarrhea and helps in gaining weight.

Spinach . . . . Very effective blood purifier; exceptional in relieving anemia and piles.

Strawberries . . . . Help reduce fever, and stimulate the flow of urine out of the body.

Sweet Potatoes . . . . Check diarrhea and help in gaining weight.

Swiss Chard . . . . Excellent nutrient source for those suffering from anemia, arthritis, acidosis.

Tomatoes . . . . Very beneficial for dyspepsia. The premiere liver food: helps purify and strengthen a weakened liver.

Turnips . . . . Good blood purifier.

Watercress. . . . . Blood purifier. Good for anemia and skin diseases.

8

How to Create
Your Individual
Vitamin/Mineral Program

Naturopaths and medical doctors both dispute the health value of supplementary vitamins: some advocate them, some do not. The common argument put forth by my fellow Naturopaths is that vitamins are not found in Nature and, hence, are not natural substances.

I certainly agree that vitamin *pills* are not found in Nature. They do not grow on trees nor spring from the earth, and so, consequently, they are not natural (although they may be made from natural compounds). Furthermore, manufactured vitamins are concentrates of nutrients at levels that do not normally exist in Nature. Yet, it is my belief, contrary to that of many orthodox Naturopaths, that vitamins do have a place in today's world.

A chemical analysis of the human body reveals that we are roughly composed of 65 percent oxygen, 18 percent carbon, 10 percent hydrogen and 3 percent nitrogen. The remaining 4 percent is a combination of minerals such as calcium, iron, potassium and iodine. Each element and mineral is important in maintaining our physical well-being. For example, potassium is an essential ingredient of red blood cells and is vital to the preservation of body flexibility and youthfulness. Deficiences of the vital minerals can cause premature aging, disease, and even death. Therefore, I prescribe mineral supplements as well as supplementary vitamins.

The minerals present in the earth cannot be directly used by man for nourishment. However, plants can assimilate minerals from the soil. When we eat fruits and vegetables, our bodies receive vital nutrients in a form they can assimilate. Although plants and certain animals can manufacture vitamins, man cannot. Therefore, man must eat plants and certain animals in order to supply his body with these essential substances.

Ideally, our foods should supply us with all the vitamins and minerals we need for life and good health. However, sadly, modern farming methods and industrial technology have adversely affected the quality of nutrients in the soil by the use of chemical fertilizers and pesticides and by widespread industrial and automobile pollution.

In addition, most of us cannot eat food freshly picked from the garden, and all too much time passes between the harvesting, shipping, storing and the preparation of food. Weeks can go by as fruits and vegetables journey from farm to kitchen. By the time a person on the East Coast eats a carrot grown in California, much of its vitamin and mineral content has been destroyed by exposure to the air. (This, unfortunately, is also true of "alive," or organically grown, foods in this country, which are usually harvested in the warm climates of California or Florida and then distributed nationwide.) The vitamin and mineral value of foods is then further depleted by improper preparation such as frying, sautéeing, boiling or reheating cooked food.

So, even though you may be eating a diet geared to your specific body and consuming organically grown products each day, I believe that vitamin and mineral supplements are necessary to supply your total nutritional requirements because most modern foods are of an inferior quality.

A blanket statement cannot be made about the supplementary vitamins any more than about proper diet. Not all bodies, for example, require more Vitamin C or pantothenic acid than is provided by their diet. Based on my years of observing the different blood types, I usually recommend that an O, who has a very active body and requires a high animal-protein diet, take vitamins B, C, E, A and D every day. He needs these additional nutrients. An A, on the other hand, who has a far less active body, needs few or no supplements because his nutritional demands are small and can be met by his diet alone.

Of course, it's impossible to make a general statement about any individual's supplementary needs. When I plan a person's supplementary program, I take into consideration many other factors such as his current physical state and his expenditure of energy. A person who is suffering with a duodenal ulcer, for example, may require Vitamin C in higher dosages than those I would usually prescribe for his blood type. Any patient with an anemic condition will usually need additional vitamins B_{12} and B_{15} plus supplementary iron tablets. A very active A may require a high-potency B-complex vitamin twice a day instead of once, or a less active O may have to reduce his stress formula (B-complex, C, E) from one a day to three a week.

When I treated a boy, aged ten, who was an A suffering with severe infections of the throat and lungs, I had to determine the strength of his constitution before I recommended his dosage of Vitamin A. While I believe that Vitamin A is essential in combating cellular infections, a type A is usually too sensitive for mega-vitamin treatment. High dosages of Vitamin A could irritate the type A's kidneys, increase the accumulation of mucus and toxicity, and thus contribute to a variety of other disorders including eczema and arthritis. After examining the boy's eyes and observing weaknesses in his kidneys and lungs, I was reluctant to recommend high-potency treatment, despite the severity of his infection.

Instead, I put the boy on a low-potency Vitamin A program (10,000 IU of A plus 400 mg Vitamin D once or twice a day) to supplement his vegetarian diet. His body responded slowly to the low dosages, but within ten days, the infection was cured without harming any other part of his body, or contributing to a future disorder.

In the following pages, I will make suggestions that will help you in determining your correct vitamin program in the same fashion that you chose your diet. Vitamin and mineral rating charts have been created for each blood type based on different levels of illness and health. Of course, without personally examining you I cannot judge absolutely which program is the one best suited to you, but I can supply you with a map to guide you. I assure you that my recommendations are safe and respectful of your individual body.

If you are only experiencing your symptoms occasionally you should begin your vitamin program at step one. Remain on the program for several months or until your symptoms begin to abate. Then, move to step two, decreasing your vitamin intake accordingly. Eventually, when your condition is healed, you can move up to step three.

If you are experiencing moderate symptoms at constant intervals, also begin your vitamin program at step one; however, take the higher recommended dosage levels. If you began your diet at level three or four, begin the vitamin program at step two, and remain at that step until your symptoms have slightly abated. At that point, move up to step three, taking the higher recommended dosages and at the more frequent intervals.

If you are not experiencing any symptoms, and your body is not fatigued or clogged with mucus, you can start your vitamin program at step two, gradually reducing your dosage to step three levels as your body experiences a heightened feeling of vitality.

(Note that I have omitted step four of the vitamin program because few people ever attain a perfect state of health on their own. A personal examination by a doctor is necessary in order to determine what vitamin program a person requires when his health has been fully restored. For this reason, I suggest that you consult a qualified Natural Healer or a medical doctor. Tell him about your disorder and your current diet, if you have not already done so. If he finds that you are completely healed you can either continue your vitamin program at step three or reduce your intake of the same vitamins to three or four times a week.)

Always remember, that in a supplementary program, as in your diet, your tenacity in adhering to a recommended program will promote the rapid improvement of your health.

TYPE A

Step One

The vitamins taken at this initial step of the program are determined by the amount of fatigue you are currently experiencing, and by the severity of your symptoms. If you are highly enervated and exhausted, and you feel a significant loss of body strength, take the highest dosage levels. If you are moderately fatigued and weakened, reduce the dosages accordingly.

There are several choices you can make in selecting B-complex vitamins. Normally I suggest that the A refrain from taking high-potency B-complex. In a low-energy body, mega-dose vitamins or high-potency stress formulas can, if taken over a period of time, create toxicity because, I believe, the large quantity of protein and nutrients in the vitamins may not be utilized or burned off. I suggest taking one low-strength B-complex three times a day. However, if you are undergoing a period of stress or emotional duress, take the high-potency stress formula (one tablet twice a day) for about a month. You should notice definite improvements in your condition after that time. Then you should switch to a weaker B-complex formula. If, however, after a month, you are still experiencing weakness and fatigue, take one high-potency stress formula and two low-potency B-complex vitamins a day, eliminating the high-potency stress formula when your condition improves.

To nourish your blood and nervous system, take 100 mg of B_{12} three to five times a day as needed. A dose of 50 mg of B_6 taken one to three times a day will be beneficial to your circulatory and nervous systems. For poor circulation, I recommend taking 50 mg of B_6 three times a day.

If you are nervous and under great stress, take 200 mg of pantothenic acid one to four times a day as required, in conjunction with the high-potency stress formula and the other B vitamins. If you are not tense and nervous, pantothenic acid, like the high-potency stress formula, should be avoided.

To help increase the amount of oxygen in your body, and to revitalize your entire system, I recommend taking 50 mg of vitamin B_{15} once or twice a day. (B_{15} has become the latest fad. Several years ago, Vitamin E was the cure-all; before that it was Vitamin C and before that, ginseng root. B_{15} is not, as is commonly believed, a new-found vitamin. Nearly fifteen years ago I was approached by a certain manufacturer to help promote it. Its chemical name is Pangamic Acid and it increases the assimilation of oxygen in the body. Inasmuch as it is a highly priced vitamin, I suggest that you be wary of a high-powered sales pitch from vitamin vendors who may proclaim it "instant healing.")

To help prevent infections and promote healthy functioning of the mucus membranes, I recommend 10,000 IU of Vitamin A, combined with 400 mg of Vitamin D (essential for growth and maintenance of normal bones and teeth) once every other day. If you are feeling exceedingly fatigued, take one or two A and D's every day.

Vitamin C, which promotes cellular activity, builds the body's defense system against disease and helps maintain the strength of the blood vessels, should be taken in small amounts by the A. I have found that large doses of Vitamin C can irritate the A's urinary tract. Recent reports by doctors Victor Herbert and Elizabeth Jacobs of Columbia University show that the very high doses of Vitamin C sometimes prescribed by doctors can destroy Vitamin B_{12} in all people and lead to pernicious anemia.

I recommend taking one 250-mg tablet of C either once a day or every other day to insure general health. If you are suffering from a respiratory condition, such as asthma, sinusitis, or chest congestion, increase the dosage to 700 to 1000 mg a day. People who smoke should also increase their intake of C because smoking destroys Vitamin C in the body. Vitamin C cannot be stored for more than a few hours in the body, so you should take precautions to insure that a deficiency does not occur. Take 250 to 1000 mg of Vitamin C a day, according to your smoking habits.

To encourage tissue repair and growth, to promote the normal functioning of the muscles and tone the nervous system, take 200 IU of Vitamin E a day. If you are tense and nervous, or have an infection, I advise increasing your intake up to 800 IU a day.

Many people today take bonemeal or dolomite to obtain their daily requirements of calcium. However, the level of phosphorus in these supplements is too strong for the A body and can have an undesirably stimulating effect on his nervous system. I recommend that you A's get your calcium from calcium lactate which has less phosphorus. Take two to five tablets a day.

To further increase the mineral content of your body I recommend that you take four to five alfalfa tablets daily. Minerals, or trace elements, serve the body in many ways. For instance, iron maintains a high quality of blood because it is one of the main components of hemoglobin, which carries oxygen from the lungs to all parts of the body. Zinc is necessary for the maintenance of muscular control in the body, and silicon, which is vital to the elasticity of the muscle of the eye, promotes healthy eyesight. Mineral deficiency plays an important part in many diseases such as arthritis, cataracts, hardening of the arteries, anemia, psoriasis and sclerosis.

To insure healthy blood and protect against anemia, take one ferrous iron tablet a day. Often, a person's stool becomes dark while taking this supplement. Don't be alarmed, the color will return to normal as your body adjusts to the additional iron.

Since I have discovered that the A, by nature, has a hyperactive thyroid, I suggest that you take three to four kelp tablets daily as a source of iodine. Iodine has a nourishing effect on the thyroid gland, helping it to form the hormone thyroxine and regulating its secretion, which controls the body's metabolism. In addition, kelp protects against the ill effects of Strontium 90 and radioactive iodine in the air released by atmospheric nuclear blasts and nuclear-power-plant leakages, such as that which occurred at the Three Mile Island plant in Pennsylvania. Some studies have shown that when kelp is absorbed by the thyroid gland it can reduce the adsorption of Strontium 90 by as much as 75 percent.

Two glutamic acid hydrochloric tablets should be taken every day to increase the acidity level in the stomach and promote better digestion. (I usually recommend this supplement to the A because I have found that the A's gastric juices tend to be deficient in hydrochloric acid and therefore do not have the high level of acidity needed to break down food particles. Glutamic acid hydrochloric is not to be confused with concentrated hydrochloric acid; it is not harmful to the body.)

To also help encourage proper digestion, you should take a digestive enzyme after every meal. The one I often recommend is a papaya-derived enzyme available at most health stores.

If you have a high level of cholesterol, I recommend that you take one to five tablespoons of lecithin (1200 IU) every day (according to the severity of your condition) to help dissolve these fatty deposits in the arteries. Sprinkle it on cereals, grains, salads or mixed vegetables.

For those suffering great fatigue, I suggest a soy protein drink several times a day. Mix one tablespoon of powder in a half a glass of water and drink before each meal (or as required) to help strengthen the body and reduce tiredness, irritability and depressions. For a minor case of fatigue, have a protein drink twice daily.

Although yeast is an excellent form of B vitamins, assists the liver in its work, and is said to protect the body against radiation, many A's have complained that yeast causes flatulence so it should therefore be avoided or used only sparingly.

Step Two

Having remained at step one for three to four months, or until a feeling of strength has been revived and certain symptoms healed, move on to step two and reduce your vitamin intake.

B-complex vitamins can now be taken once or twice a day. Low-potency formulas are recommended. Take the high-potency stress formula only during periods of extreme tension or stress.

Since your nervous system has been nourished and calmed, you may now reduce your B_{12} intake to 100 mg two or three times a day. Fifty mg of B_6 can now be taken once or twice a day as your circulatory and nervous systems improve, and B_{15} can be reduced to one a day.

Ten thousand IU of Vitamin A and 400 mg of Vitamin D should be continued at the same level of one a day. Take 250 to 1000 mg of Vitamin C once a day (the dosage to be determined by your current respiratory condition and the amount of cigarettes you are still smoking).

Vitamin E should be taken in doses ranging from 200 to 800 IU a day, depending upon the state of your nervous system and/or the severity of any infections in your body.

Four to five alfalfa tablets should be taken every day to provide vital minerals. Calcium lactate tablets can be reduced to two to three tablets a day as energy levels improve. (A reduction of nervous energy would indicate that your thyroid gland has been normalizing and that the metabolic rate is slowing down.) Ferrous iron can now be reduced to one a day.

Glutamic acid hydrochloric tablets should be taken once a day to insure proper digestive activity in your stomach. Now, the papaya-derived enzymes can be reduced to two a day, following lunch and dinner.

Lecithin (1200 IU) can be reduced according to a decrease in your cholesterol count or improvement in vascular conditions (this should be determined by your doctor) to one to three tablespoons a day.

As fatigue is replaced by increased feelings of vitality, reduce the soy protein drink to once or twice a day, according to your energy needs.

Step Three

It can take the A a long time to reach an ideal state of health when few or no vitamins are necessary. These are my recommendations for the state of health most A's attain after my treatment.

B-complex can now be reduced to one a day and 100 mg of B_{12} and 50 mg of B_6 can be taken once a day. Ten thousand IU of Vitamin A and 400 mg of Vitamin D, 250 mg of Vitamin C and 200 IU of Vitamin E should be taken every other day.

Glutamic acid hydrochloric tablets should be taken once a day and a papaya-derived digestive enzyme should now only be taken once a day, following the heaviest meal.

B_{15} and ferrous iron are no longer required. Lecithin (1200 IU) can be eliminated when cholesterol levels have been normalized, and when fatigue is no longer a problem, you may stop drinking soy protein.

Although types A, B and AB will eventually reduce their vitamin intake to the levels suggested in step three, those individuals with type-O blood will always require more vitamin supplementation because of their high energy and nutritional requirements. Therefore there are only two steps in the O's vitamin program instead of the three-step program recommended for the other groups.

TYPE O

Step One

To determine an O's vitamin program, one must consider his current physical condition and the amount of energy he expends.

If you are very active and tend to burn off a lot of energy, you will need high-dosage vitamins. If you are a less active O, less supplementation will be required.

134

Because O's usually are energetic people, they should take two or three high-potency stress complex formulas a day.

To nourish muscles and nerves, take B_{12} (500 mg) two or three times a day, and to stimulate blood circulation and encourage protein and carbohydrate metabolism, take B_6 in 50-mg dosages three times a day.

For the proper functioning of your heart, nerves and muscles, and to assist in carbohydrate metabolism, take vitamins B_1 and B_2 in 50-mg dosages one to three times a day (according to the amount of your physical energy). If in the past you have had rheumatic fever or a coronary thrombosis with resultant damage to heart tissue, I recommend that you increase the dosage level to 100 mg and take three a day.

Vitamins A and D should be taken together once or twice a day as needed: 25,000 IU of Vitamin A and 1000 mg of Vitamin D. If you have skin or mucous-membrane irritations, such as eczema or chest congestion, and are an adult, take three A and D a day (children and the elderly should restrict their intake to one a day). Vitamin E should be taken in 400-IU doses two or three times a day according to your body's need for tissue repair. Vitamin C should be taken in doses ranging from 500 to 3000 mg every day, based on the number of cigarettes you are smoking, your vulnerability to illness or the presence of such respiratory disorders as asthma, sinusitis, pneumonia or bronchitis.

If you are under great stress, take pantothenic acid in 200-mg dosages, one to six times a day as needed.

To help meet your daily requirement of calcium, which is vital to the health of your teeth, gums and skeletal system, take one to six tablets of bonemeal or dolomite every day as your condition requires.

To increase the minerals in your body, take one to ten alfalfa tablets a day, and to improve your red-blood-cell count or help heal anemic conditions take ferrous iron once or twice a day.

O's with high-cholesterol counts should take from one to five tablespoons of lecithin (1200 IU) a day.

When fatigue is present, one of the following programs should be instituted. If you feel mildly fatigued, mix one-and-a-half tablespoons of soy protein powder into a half-a-glass of water and drink three to five times a day. If your body feels really run-down and tired, and you suffer from depression and irritability, I recommend that you mix a tablespoon of liquid protein in a glass of water and drink this five times a day.

Recent reports have condemned the use of liquid protein, because of its dangerous side effects which have in a few cases been fatal. I am in total agreement with the FDA: liquid protein can be *highly dangerous to the body,* but only under certain circumstances.

I believe that for a person with small protein requirements, such as a type A or AB, liquid protein, which is a high concentrate of protein nutrients, can tax and possibly irritate the digestive system. Without a doubt the entire system comes under undue stress as it tries to assimilate the excessive amount of nutrients. The nervous system is strained by the increased stress on the body, and all unused proteins, I believe, are transformed into toxic wastes. Fatigue may overcome the body because of this internal disharmony causing a variety of mental disorders including severe depressions and confusion. This can occur in all blood types, and it invariably happens when the body is not receiving other types of foods.

In cases where adverse side effects resulted, all other foods had been virtually eliminated from the person's diet. Because of the lack of properly balanced meals, the high concentration of proteins disturbed the electrolyte balance and very probably shocked the digestive system, which had been accustomed to receiving daily allowances of many kinds of nutrients and now had to break down an unusually large amount of protein alone. In these cases of sudden death, the killer was not the liquid protein but the lack of other nutrients: people actually starved themselves to death.

The body cannot sustain severe shock by drastic dietary changes. One may lose ten to twenty pounds within days by going on this kind of diet, but you can bet that if a side effect does not occur immediately, the diet has significantly contributed to the production of a future disorder.

Used under the conditions I recommend—in conjunction with a balanced diet, and only for a short period of time—liquid protein can be a beneficial supplement. The body is not shocked by the sudden increase of protein and reduction of other foodstuff; instead it receives all its required nutrients and is allowed to regain its well-being gradually without shock or distress. Even though there are several chemicals included in the liquid-protein formula, I have found, in case after case, that this supplement helps the body to regenerate its vitality without harmful side effects. Of course people argue, "It's not natural." Again, I agree. But there are times when I must choose to prescribe a food or supplement which, although not completely organic, will do more good than harm. As I have said, we live in today's world, and part of coping with a world that is highly polluted and chemically oriented is weighing one's options in order to recommend foods or supplements that will provide the best health in the most responsible fashion.

Therefore, I recommend that as the body regains its energy, the soy protein powder or liquid protein drink be reduced to three times a day.

During this period, take one papaya-derived digestive enzyme after every meal to help facilitate proper digestion.

Step Two

After three or four months, or as your body regains its strength and begins to feel revitalized, reduce your vitamin levels.

The high-potency stress-B-complex formula can now be reduced to one or two tablets a day. Take one B_{12} (500 mg), one B_6 (50 mg), and one B_1 and B_2 (50 mg) every day. B_{15} can now be reduced to one a day.

Ten thousand IU Vitamin A, 500 mg Vitamin D, 400 IU Vitamin E and 500 to 2000 mg Vitamin C should now be taken daily.

Bonemeal or dolomite can be reduced to three tablets a day, and alfalfa to one to seven tablets every day.

If your cholesterol count has been lessened, reduce your intake of lecithin (1200 IU) to one or two tablespoons a day.

Ferrous iron should be taken once a day, and the soy protein or liquid protein drink can now be reduced to once or twice a day, as required.

The papaya-derived enzyme can now be reduced to twice a day, one after lunch and one after dinner.

If you are still very stressed or tense, take 200 mg of pantothenic acid twice a day.

Follow this program for six to eight months.

Because the ideal state of health can take a long time to reach, the following are my recommendations for the state of health that most O's who have been through this program attain.

Take one high-potency stress-B-complex formula, plus 500 mg of B_{12}, 50 mg of B_6 and one B_{15} tablet once a day.

Vitamin A (25,000 IU and Vitamin D (1000 mg), Vitamin E (400 IU) and Vitamin C (500 mg) should also be taken once a day.

One or two 50-mg tablets of B_1 and B_2 should be taken every other day.

If you still have stress and tension, take 200 mg of pantothenic acid every day as long as the condition persists. Ferrous iron should be taken once a day, bonemeal or dolomite twice a day and alfalfa tablets five times a day.

If your cholesterol count has been lowered to a normal level, eliminate lecithin, and if fatigue is no longer a problem, you may stop drinking soy protein or liquid protein.

The papaya-derived digestive enzyme should now be taken once a day, following the heaviest meal of the day.

TYPE B

Step One

Because type B's are midway between A and O, your vitamin regimen, like your diet, will be determined by either your energy

138

level or the concentration of mucus in your body. If you are experiencing fatigue and a low-energy level, follow a vitamin program similar to type O; if you are catarrhal in nature, lean toward the type-A program.

If you are a B with a catarrhal nature and suffer any of the catarrhal-related illnesses such as arthritis, bronchitis, chest congestion or sinusitis, follow this program as your step one.

In order to tone and strengthen your body, take one low-potency B-complex vitamin three times a day. If you also feel slightly run-down or fatigued, combine the low-potency vitamin with a high-potency stress formula. Take two low-potency B-complex tablets and one high-potency stress formula a day.

To nourish your circulatory and nervous systems, take 100 mg of B_{12} four to six times a day. To help promote a healthy nervous system and improve the functioning of your muscles, take 50 mg of B_6 two or three times a day.

Ten thousand IU of Vitamin A and 400 mg of Vitamin D should be taken twice a day. Increase this dosage to three or four times a day if you have severe skin irritations, a susceptibility to infection, disorders of the eye, or catarrhal-related illnesses such as arthritis, bronchitis or pneumonia.

Two hundred IU of Vitamin E should be taken from one to four times a day depending upon your need for tissue repair and general vitality.

Your Vitamin C intake may be greater than that of an A because your tolerance for this vitamin is greater. You can start with 250 mg a day, and increase the dosage as high as 2000 mg a day, according to the severity of your disorder. For sore, bleeding gums and loose teeth for instance, I advise 1000 to 2000 mg until the condition abates. If you have a tendency to bruise easily, I advise 750 to 1000 mg a day; for sinus problems or susceptibility to colds or the flu, 1500 mg a day (children and elderly people should take about half the dosage of an adult).

If you are suffering with anemia, brittleness of the hair, sagging skin, loss of muscular strength, boils, or other symptoms of toxicity in the body, take one to seven alfalfa tablets a day according to the severity of your condition. Increasing such minerals as copper, manganese and silicon in the body will gradually rebuild your weakened tissues and muscles and, I have found, help cleanse waste and morbid matter from your body.

To help meet your calcium requirement, take one to five tablets of calcium lactate or dolomite daily. (B's, unlike A's, are not adversely affected by the concentration of phosphorus in the dolomite.)

If you are anemic or feeling sluggish, take ferrous iron once a day. (A reminder: Ferrous iron can turn your stool a dark reddish-brown and possibly cause constipation; continue taking because this condition will soon stop.) In addition, include a soy protein drink in your daily program. Mix one-and-a-half table-spoons of soy protein powder in a half-a-glass of water and drink one to five times a day as needed.

If you have a cholesterol buildup, take one to three tablespoons of lecithin (1200 IU) every day. Sprinkle this on your cereals, grains or salads.

Following each meal, take a papaya-derived enzyme to facilitate better digestion.

Stay on this program for three to six months, or until you can feel that the concentrations of catarrh have been broken up and there is a distinct change in your condition.

If you are a B suffering from great fatigue, with such accompanying symptoms as lethargy and depressions, lean toward the O regimen and follow this program as your step one.

To reduce fatigue and strengthen your body, take two high-potency stress formulas and one low-potency B-complex tablet every day. In addition, 100 mg of B_{12} should be taken four to six times a day, and 50 mg of B_6 three times a day. To help regenerate your energy, vitamins B_1 and B_2 should be introduced in dosages of 50 mg twice a day. These vitamins have a tendency to create gas in type B's, so carefully monitor your body's reactions within the first few days of adding these vitamins to your program. If gas should occur, reduce your intake of B_1 and B_2 to one a day. If the condition persists, try eliminating them altogether and see if the gas stops. If it does, forego taking these vitamins. If the gas persists, the vitamins are probably not the cause and you can resume taking them.

Ten thousand IU of Vitamin A and 400 mg of Vitamin D should be taken once a day. Two hundred IU of Vitamin E should be taken one to four times a day, depending upon your need to increase your body's vitality or heal infections. Vitamin C can be taken in 250-mg dosages three to four times a day. If you are experiencing mental lulls and apathy along with your fatigue, are very susceptible to colds and the flu, or are now smoking a lot, you can increase your intake up to 2000 mg a day.

To increase the minerals in your body, take one to seven alfalfa tablets a day. If your fatigue or loss of strength is caused by an anemic condition, take the maximum dosage, and to heighten your general body strength take from one to five a day.

If your fatigue is mild, mix one-and-a-half tablespoons of soy protein powder in a half-a-glass of water and drink one to five times a day, whenever you feel a sudden loss of energy. In cases of excessive fatigue, the B should take the soy protein drink twice a day plus one tablespoon of liquid protein mixed in a half-a-glass of water twice a day. This will speed the regeneration of your body's vitality.

To meet your calcium requirements, take one to five tablets of dolomite or calcium lactate as required. B's with cholesterol deposits should mix one to three tablespoons of lecithin (1200 IU) with salads or grains.

To help stimulate your blood, take one tablet of ferrous iron a day, and to aid digestion, I recommend one papaya-derived digestive enzyme after every meal.

This program should be followed for three to six months, or until fatigue has disappeared and you feel consistently strong and vital. Do not stop the program with the *first* feeling of renewed vitality. A fatigued body will be energized within days after starting the program, but any body that has been run-down and weakened has to be rebuilt gradually—and this will take time.

Step Two

B Catarrhal nature: Low-potency B-complex vitamins should now be taken twice a day; 100 mg of B_{12} three times a day, and 50 mg of B_6 twice a day.

Continue taking 10,000 IU Vitamin A and 400 mg of Vitamin D twice a day to repair and soothe irritated or inflamed mucous membranes in the lungs or kidneys or to clear up skin eruptions. Take 200 IU of Vitamin E one to three times a day (as required), and up to 2000 mg Vitamin C a day, the amount determined by your susceptibility to colds, smoking habits, or the degree of your congestion.

Now, you may reduce your daily dosage to four or five alfalfa tablets and three or four calcium lactate or dolomites.

If your mild fatigue has been controlled, reduce your intake of the soy protein drink to twice a day. If your cholesterol count has been lowered, you can reduce lecithin to one or two tablespoons daily.

Ferrous iron can now be taken once every other day, unless anemic conditions persist. If there is anemia, continue taking iron once a day.

The papaya-derived digestive enzyme can now be reduced to two a day, one after lunch and one after dinner.

Fatigued B: As fatigue decreases and energy levels rise, reduce the high-potency stress formula to one a day. In addition, take one low-potency B-complex every day. When you are no longer run-down and enervated you may eliminate the high-potency stress formula but take the low-potency B-complex twice a day.

One hundred mg of B_{12} can now be taken two or three times a day, and 50 mg of B_6 may also be reduced to twice a day. If your strength has been greatly improved, and you do not have excessive gas, reduce vitamins B_1 and B_2 to one each day or eliminate them.

Take 10,000 IU of Vitamin A, 400 mg of Vitamin D once a day, and 200 IU of Vitamin E once or twice a day. Vitamin C should be continued in dosages ranging from 250 to 2000 mg

142

according to your susceptibility to colds, mucus irritations and the amount of cigarettes you are still smoking.

Three calcium lactate or dolomite tablets and four alfalfa tablets should be taken daily. Lecithin can be reduced to one or two tablespoons a day if your cholesterol count has been lowered.

Ferrous iron can now be taken once every other day unless you still experience periods of sudden weakness, which will be helped by a daily dosage of iron.

During this period excessive fatigue will be replaced by a consistent feeling of strength and well-being, and as midday lulls or the need for catnaps are reduced, cut your consumption of the soy protein to one to three times a day. The liquid-protein combination can now be reduced to one a day. The papaya-derived digestive enzyme should be taken twice a day, following lunch and dinner.

Follow this program for four to six months to insure that your body fully regenerates its strength and energy.

Step Three

By this stage, both catarrhal and fatigued conditions should be stabilized. Most B's who have been through the program now follow this regimen.

Take one or two low-potency B-complex vitamins a day, according to your energy requirements. If you have a physically demanding job, or you are nervous or under stress, take one low-potency and one high-potency stress formula a day. One or two 100 mg of vitamin B_{12}, and one 50 mg of vitamin B_6 should also be taken every day.

Ten thousand IU of Vitamin A and 400 mg of Vitamin D, 200 IU of Vitamin E and 250 mg of Vitamin C should be taken every other day. (You can increase your intake of Vitamin C to 500 to 750 mg a day in cold weather to build your body's resistance, or if you are still smoking.)

Two alfalfa and two calcium-lactate or dolomite tablets should be taken daily. Ferrous iron can now be reduced to one a week.

143

The soy protein and liquid protein drinks and the lecithin (1200 IU) can all be eliminated.

One papaya-derived digestive enzyme should be taken after the heavy meal of the day to encourage proper digestion and assimilation of nutrients.

TYPE AB

Step One

Because type AB's have characteristics closely related to those of the type A and follow a similar diet, their vitamin program is based on the A regimen.

The AB should take one low-potency B-complex vitamin three times a day. High-potency stress formulas should be taken during periods of emotional duress, but only for brief periods. If these vitamins are taken for an extended amount of time, I have found that the excessive nutrients will be converted into toxicity within the body, thus defeating their purpose.

To nourish and soothe your nervous system, take 100 mg of B_{12} three to five times a day, and 50 mg of B_6 three to five times a day. AB's experiencing stress or tension should also take 200 mg of pantothenic acid one to four times a day as needed.

To heighten the amount of oxygen in your body and hasten its utilization, take one or two B_{15} a day.

Take 10,000 IU of Vitamin A and 400 mg of Vitamin D once every other day to promote health and proper functioning of your mucous membranes. When you have mucus congestion, take the vitamins A and D every day to help soothe the irritated membrane lining.

Take 200 IU of Vitamin E every day. If you are suffering with tissue damage, infections or catarrhal conditions, increase your Vitamin E to 800 IU a day.

Your Vitamin C intake should be limited, because I have found that it can irritate your urinary tract and also cause stomach cramps if taken in mega-dosages. A dose of 250 mg a day will help maintain your body's resistance against illness and contribute to the health of your blood vessels. However, those AB's who have an irritation of the mucous membranes (asthma or arthritis) or who are still smoking should increase Vitamin C to 700 to 1000 mg a day.

To introduce minerals into your body, take four to five alfalfa tablets each day, and to meet your daily requirements of calcium, take two to five tablets of calcium lactate daily.

Avoid taking dolomite and bonemeal because their high phosphorus level can have a stimulating effect on your already highly active nervous system.

To insure healthy blood and protect against anemia and fatigue, take ferrous iron once a day. As I have discovered that the AB is, by nature, hyperactive (owing to a slight abnormality of the thyroid gland), you should take one to four tablets of kelp a day to regulate thyroid hormone secretion. Kelp tablets are recommended because they have higher concentrations of iodine than are to be found in seaweed in its natural state.

If you suffer from fatigue, take one-and-a-half tablespoons of soy protein powder (available in most health stores) in a half-a-glass of water four to five times a day according to your energy requirements.

To increase the acidity level in your stomach and promote proper digestion, take one glutamic-acid hydrochloric tablet once a day. (This is not to be confused with concentrated hydrochloric acid; glutamic-acid hydrochloric tablets are not harmful to the body.) A papaya-derived digestive enzyme should also be taken following each meal.

If you have cholesterol or other vascular fat deposits, take a tablespoon of lecithin (1200 IU) one to five times a day according to the severity of your condition.

The AB will experience gas when digesting brewer's yeast and should therefore either avoid it or use it sparingly.

Step Two

Remain at step one for three to four months, or until a feeling

145

of strength has been revived and certain symptoms healed, then move to step three and reduce your vitamin intake.

The low-potency B-complex vitamin can now be taken once or twice a day as required; 100 mg of Vitamin B_{12} two to three times a day and 50 mg of B_6 can be taken once or twice daily.

Take 10,000 IU of Vitamin A, 400 mg of Vitamin D, 200 IU of Vitamin E and 250 to 1000 mg of Vitamin C only once a day.

Four alfalfa and three calcium-lactate tablets should be taken daily, and as you experience a lowered level of nervous energy, kelp can be reduced to two or three a day.

As cholesterol levels are lowered (this will have to be determined by your doctor), you may reduce your intake of lecithin to one to three tablespoons a day according to your needs. When your energy level has been increased and your fatigue lessened, reduce your soy protein drink to once or twice a day.

Glutamic-acid hydrochloric tablets and ferrous iron should be taken once a day. Now, the papaya-derived digestive enzyme can be reduced to two a day, one after lunch and one after dinner.

This step should be followed for six to eight months.

Step Three

Because it will take a person with type-AB blood a long time to reach an ideal state of health, when few or no vitamins will be required, these are my recommendations for a vitamin program geared to the state of health most AB's will attain after following steps one and two.

Take one low-potency B-complex, 100 mg of B_{12} and 50 mg of B_6 once a day.

Take 10,000 IU of Vitamin A and 400 mg of Vitamin D, 200 IU of Vitamin E and 250 mg of Vitamin C each once every other day.

Calcium lactate should be reduced to two a day, kelp to one a day and alfalfa to three a day.

Glutamic-acid hydrochloric tablets should be continued once a day, ferrous iron should be taken once a week, and one papaya-derived digestive enzyme should be taken following the heaviest meal of the day.

Lecithin (1200 IU) and the soy protein drink can be eliminated.

No regimen should be inflexible. For instance, you may go off your diet and cause a disorder in your body, or overwork and suffer severe mental stress. Traveling, changing occupations, family problems—any event which alters the normal course of your life—can affect your health and necessitate a change in your dietary and vitamin requirements.

You may find you must temporarily return to a previous step, increase the dosage of high-potency stress formula vitamins to help you cope with an emotional problem, or take additional Vitamin C if your resistance is lowered and you have contracted a cold or the flu.

Remember, these programs are only suggestions. You may want, after careful consideration, to add a supplement according to a need I have not discussed, perhaps taking vegetal silica to improve brittle nails. However, this should not be in response to a suggestion by your health food store owner or a druggist who may want to sell a vitamin with which he is overstocked. Before you add to my program, consult a Natural Healer, or your medical doctor.

Vitamin programs today are a dime a dozen. Adele Davis tells you one thing, *Prevention* magazine another and medical doctors or professional science nutritionists still something else. At some point *you* are going to have to contribute in deciding what is right for you.

If your supplementary program is balanced by a good sound diet and your dosage levels are moderate (remember all my recommendations are specific for each blood type), you can be assured that you will not be creating toxicity in your body through "nutritional overdose."

VITAL MINERALS

Mineral	Health Value	Sources
Calcium	Builds bones and teeth, essential in normal clotting of blood and for proper growth. Promotes normal responses of muscles and nerves.	Asparagus, beans, cauliflower, beets, cabbage, carrots, celery, dairy products, kale, almonds, greens
Cobalt	Forms part of Vitamin B_{12}. Essential in the prevention of anemia and rheumatic diseases.	Liver, leafy vegetables, fish, whole cereals, legumes
Copper	Helps in the formation of hemoglobin.	Bran, liver, mushrooms, peas, leafy vegetables, nuts, fish, poultry, whole grains
Iodine	Promotes health of the thyroid gland. Essential to metabolism.	Fish, sea plants, bran broccoli, butter, carrots, spinach, cherries, corn, and oats
Iron	Promotes the development of red blood cells. Principal component of hemoglobin.	Almonds, asparagus, beans, kale, cauliflower, celery, chard, dandelion, egg yolk, hearts, kidneys, liver, fish, currants, oranges and poultry
Magnesium	Essential to bones, muscular activities, the nervous system and the brain. Activates digestive enzymes.	Almonds, barley, chard, beans, corn, peas, potatoes, fish, watercress, carrots, dandelion
Manganese	Promotes growth and is necessary to a healthy reproductive system.	Beans, beets, bran, chard, peas, leafy greens, whole grains, almonds
Nickel	Helps the body digest sugar.	Beansprouts, lettuce, onions, garlic, seaweed, celery, string beans

Mineral	Health value	Sources
Phosphorus	Combines with calcium to build bone. Helps maintain alkalinity of the blood. Necessary for the digestion of carbohydrates and fats.	Almonds, barley, beans, bran, eggs, cheese, lentils, liver, milk, fish, whole wheat, corn, and peas
Potassium	Essential ingredient of the blood, the brain and nerve cells.	Beans, bran, olives, potatoes, spinach, beets, cabbage, celery, lettuce, parsnips
Sulphur	Necessary for the proper functioning of the nerves. Helps the body build cells.	Beans, cheese, eggs, fish, lean meats, peas, chard, oats, watercress and onions
Sodium	Maintains osmotic pressure: the balance of pressure in blood vessels, lymph glands and tissues.	Cheese, beets, carrots, chard, watercress, wheatgerm, spinach, olives, eggs and turnips
Silicon	Necessary for the proper growth of hair, nails and teeth.	Fruits with skin, whole wheat, peas, asparagus, endives, figs, carrots, beets, cherries, tomatoes
Zinc	Sparks vitamin activity, aids tissue respiration, necessary for correct insulin function.	Beans, watercress, dandelion, peas, liver, lentils, fish, broccoli, spinach

MINERAL VALUE OF HERBS

The lack of organic salts such as potassium, sodium, iron and iodine is often a contributing cause of various bodily ills. Replacing these organic substances through the use of herbal teas can help the body build up its resistance and combat disease. The following groups of herbs are helpful in various conditions.

ONE MAN'S FOOD . . .

Potassium-Rich Herbs

Herbs	Used for
Oak Bark	Diseases of the lungs and chest
Comfrey	Liver and spleen disorders
Yarrow	Regulating the bowels
Primrose Flowers;	The functioning of brain and nervous system
Summer Savory	
American Centaury	Insomnia and acid stomach
Plantain Leaves;	Strengthening the heart muscles
Mullein	

Sodium-Rich Herbs

Herbs	Used for
Apple Tree Bark	Hardening of the arteries
Huckleberry Leaves	Diabetes
Fennel Seed	Gallstones
Shepherd's Purse	Arthritis
Anise Seed	Bladder stones
Black Willow	Rheumatism
Cleavers	Acid-mucus-condition
Stinging Nettle;	Retard aging
Mistletoe; Dill	

Calcium-Rich Herbs

Herbs		Used for
Horsetail	Mistletoe	Bone and teeth conditions
Plantain; Nettles	Cleavers; Watercress	Pregnant women (especially the last three months)
Dandelion	Dill	Impoverished blood
Pimpernel	Toadflax	Asthma
Meadowsweet	Chives	Hemorrhages
Poppy Seed		Corpulency
Chamomile		Strengthening heart muscles
Rest Harrow		Building the body structure
Caraway Seed		Increasing resistance

150

Herbs
Silverweed;
Tormentil
root; Colts-
foot; Shep-
herd's Purse

Used for
Valuable in all children's diseases

Magnesium-Rich Herbs

Herbs		*Used for*
Carrot Leaves	Silverweed	Arrest and prevent tooth decay
Meadowsweet	Devil's Bit	Insomnia and irritability
Mistletoe	Rest Harrow	Poor circulation and im-
Mullein Leaves	Toadflax	poverished blood
Broom Tops	Nettles	Nervous prostration
Walnut Leaves		Tuberculosis, chest diseases
Dill; Primrose; Black Willow Bark		Low resistance

Iron-Rich Herbs

Herbs		*Used for*
Acorns, sweet	Strawberry lvs	Anemia (chlorosis)
Sorrel; Nettles	Chives; Dandelion	Strengthen "power station" (spleen)
Poppy Seed	Irish Moss	Prevent weakness in old age
Yellow Dock	Burdock	Strengthens the liver
Huckleberry Leaves	Silverweed	Shortness of breath
Stinging Nettles	Devil's Bit	Greater physical and mental power
Salep; Mullein Leaves	Meadowsweet; Rest Harrow	Extending the lifespan

Copper-Rich Herbs

Herbs	*Used for*
Agar-agar	Chronic indigestion
Liverwort	Gallbladder disorders

151

Herbs		Used for
Sea Oak		Diabetes (pancreas). See Nickel-Rich Herbs
Sorrel		Liver (bile secretion)
Choy		Child growth (Thymus secretion)
Kelp		Normal sex glands
Limu		Bone adjustment
Nettles		Low blood pressure
Dulse		Spleen
Salep		Goiter (see Iodine-Rich Herbs)
Devil's Bit; Dandelion		Scanty urine

Nickel-Rich Herbs

Herbs		Used for
Choy; Limu; Liverwort; Kelp	Algae; Bladder Wrack	Regulates blood sugar

Phosphorus-Rich Herbs

Herbs		Used for
Rhubarb Calamus	Marigold Flowers; Licorice Root	Strengthen the Nerves (especially of the heart)
Watercress	Chickweed	Nervous indigestion
Meadowsweet; Dill	Sorrel	Brain development for psychic and metaphysical work; electric brain and nerve impulses; general bodily poise; normal sex power; neuritis; hypochondria

Sulphur-Rich Herbs

Herbs		Used for
Scouring Rush	Eyebright	Dissolves the acids in system
Mullein	Rest Harrow	Antiseptic for alimentary canal
Meadowsweet	Fennel	Warms body and feet

152

Herbs		Used for
Plantain Leaves	Stinging Nettle	Energy and high spirits
Shepherd's Purse	Silverweed	Strengthens the tissues
Waywort	Broom Tops	Beautify the skin and hair
Coltsfoot	Pimpernel	Pep and personality

Manganese-Rich Herbs

Herbs		Used for
Kelp; Dulse	Strawberry Leaves; Wintergreen	Increase gland secretion
Agar-agar	Yellow Dock	Reducing
Choy	Burdock	Pregnant and nursing mothers
Limu	Stinging Nettle	Mental alertness
Sea Wrack		Neuritis
Sorrel		Fortitude in shock and sorrow; Poor eyesight from mental strain; Neurasthenia

Silicon-Rich Herbs

Herbs		Used for
Lamb's Lettuce	Cornsilk	Diabetes
Red Raspberry Leaves	Sunflower Seeds	Prevent Infection
Chickweed	Poppy Seed	Blood diseases and poor circulation
Flaxseed		Soft bones and teeth; nervous exhaustion; loss of hair and ridged nails; failing eyesight; sensitivity to drafts

Chlorine-Rich Herbs

Herbs		Used for
Bearberry	Plantain	Sinus trouble

153

Herbs		Used for
Mistletoe	Watercress;	Bright's disease
Stems; Fennel	Limu	
Stems		
Dill Stems		Adjusting weight
Myrrh		Stiff joints
Wintergreen		Pyorrhea, bloated abdomen, gastric and other secretions, repairing the organs, enriching the blood

Fluorine-Rich Herbs

Herbs	Used for
Cornsilk	Weakened eyesight
Watercress	Curvature of the spine
Dill	Early decay of children's teeth
Horsetail	Skin disorders
Plantain	Arrests the processes of decay
Grain-coats	Repairing broken bones, developing the bony structure of the body

Iodine-Rich Herbs

Herbs	Used for
Sea Wrack	Goiter
Irish Moss;	Assists before and during childbirth
Iceland Moss	
Mustard;	Retaining the natural color of the hair
Algae	
Kelp;	Proper development during adolescence
Parsley	
Nettles	Obesity (disposes of fats)
Dulse	Mental fortitude and healthy nerves

Based on the teaching of Sebastian Kneipp

VITAMIN VALUE OF FOODS
VITAMIN A

Primary sources are green and yellow vegetables, certain fruits and dairy products, and animal liver. Since Vitamin A is not water soluble, cooking does not destroy the Vitamin A content of vegetables. The following foods are excellent sources of this essential vitamin: apricots (fresh or dried), broccoli, cantaloupe, carrots, celery, cabbage, chard, cheese, collards, dandelion greens, endive, kale, lettuce (green), calf's liver, mustard greens, parsley, peaches (fresh and dried), spinach, squash (winter), sweet potatoes, turnip greens and watercress.

Note: White vegetables such as cauliflower, cucumbers, white potatoes, turnips and white onions have virtually no Vitamin A.

VITAMIN B-COMPLEX

The B-complex consists of thiamine, riboflavin, niacin, pantothenic acid, pyridoxine, choline, inositol, Vitamin B_{12}, biotin and para-amino-benzoic acid (PABA). These vitamins are found mainly in the outer husk of seeds and cereals—and are completely lacking in bleached flour and polished rice. Other sources of B vitamins include: yeast, fruit, vegetables, nuts, meat, fish and milk. These foods contain plentiful amounts of the various B vitamins: asparagus, beans (fresh and dried), buckwheat, brewer's yeast, cabbage, corn, celery, mustard greens, nuts—almonds, filberts (hazelnuts), peanuts—ryegerm, soy beans, spinach, tangerines, turnip greens, watercress and wheatgerm. Animal and dairy sources include cheese, eggs, liver, milk, and veal.

Note: The B vitamins are all water soluble. Therefore, if you discard the water in which meat and vegetables have been cooked—you throw the B vitamins away.

VITAMIN C

The best sources of Vitamin C are the citrus fruits: orange, tangerine, grapefruit, lemon and lime. Both the pulp and the peel of these fruits contain large amounts of Vitamin C (ascorbic acid). Other foods rich in Vitamin C include: apples, blueberries, Brussels sprouts, cabbage, cantaloupe, carrots, celery, chard, cranberries, endive, peas, peppers, pineapple, rhubarb, spinach, tomatoes, turnip greens and watercress.

Note: Vitamin C is water soluble and is best obtained by eating fresh fruits or by drinking freshly made fruit juices.

VITAMIN D

This vitamin, which is essential for proper bone and tooth formation and growth, is fat soluble. The highest concentration of Vitamin D is found in fish-liver oils. Eggs, butter, fish and meat are also good sources of Vitamin D. There is virtually no Vitamin D in vegetables, cereals and fruits.

Note: The human body is its own "Vitamin D factory." When skin is exposed to sunlight, the ultraviolet rays convert a substance (7-dehydro-cholesterol) in the human skin to Vitamin D.

VITAMIN E

Vitamin E (tocopherol) is a fat soluble vitamin found chiefly in the germ oil of cereals (wheat, corn, soy, sunflower, etc.). Other foods that contain significant amounts of Vitamin E are cauliflower, spinach, kale, Brussels sprouts, milk and cheese.

VITAMIN K

Vitamin K is a fat soluble substance which is necessary for normal blood clotting. The requirement for this vitamin is extremely small. Vitamin K may be obtained from vegetable oils and from most leafy green vegetables.

VITAMIN M

This vitamin, which is usually called folic acid, is essential to the manufacture of red blood corpuscles. Folic acid occurs in nearly all foods, but the richest sources are yeast, liver, and fresh green vegetables.

Note: As much as 95 percent of the folic-acid content of foods can be destroyed by canning or long cooking. Therefore, this essential vitamin should be obtained from uncooked vegetables such as lettuce, celery, green peppers, spinach, etc.

VITAMIN P

This vitamin, also called flavonoid, is largely concentrated in the peel and pulp of citrus fruits. The value of this vitamin in human nutrition has not yet been established, although it is known that Vitamin P assists the activity of Vitamin C

9

The Art of Eating

Up to this point, I have discussed the importance of eating the right foods. As I have emphasized, food is fuel for the body, but *proper* eating entails more than simply choosing foods harmonious with your body. The way food is digested is also a vital determinant of the nutritional benefits you receive.

Sitting Pretty, a movie made in the late forties, illustrates what I mean by proper eating. The actor, Clifton Webb, portrayed Mr. Belvedere, a male nanny hired to subdue three rambunctious boys, aged two, six and ten. On his first morning at the breakfast table, Mr. Belvedere instructed the boys in the right way to eat. "Sit in silence and chew your porridge and toast seventy-five times. Not fifty, fifty-five or sixty-five, but seventy-five times," he bellowed with the ferocity of a Marine drill-sergeant.

Awed and frightened by the stern-faced disciplinarian, the two older boys obeyed the orders. Their baby brother, however, continued to gulp and incorrigibly gurgle his porridge. When the infant playfully flung a spoon of piping-hot cereal at Mr. Belvedere's face, the nanny reacted by dumping the rest of the bowl on the boy's head. Though hysterical, the child learned his lesson and in subsequent scenes, he ate quietly.

This, of course, is a rather severe way to teach correct eating habits, and certainly not one that I would recommend. However, Mr. Belvedere was not really mistaken in the practice he was trying to instill in the boys.

Eating is an art. A bon vivant dining on haute cuisine with an expensive bottle of wine is not practicing the art of eating. The true art of eating, though certainly less glamorous, is vitally important to your health. It consists of thoroughly digesting your food so that all the nutrients, including the amino acids, vitamins and minerals, can be assimilated into your body. Only food that is completely broken down into its smallest particles can be absorbed by your blood and distributed to all parts of your body.

Knowing *how* to eat, as well as *what* to eat, is what I am going to explore in this chapter.

Several factors are essential to healthy digestion. These include: eating in silence, masticating your food thoroughly, knowing when and how much to eat and which foods to combine at the same meal. Before I elaborate on these practices, let me quickly define digestion as a complex operation in which all organs of the alimentary tract secrete enzymes, catalytic agents that activate the biochemic decomposition of food substances preparing them for assimilation. There are enzymatic particles in every cell of the body, and different enzymes break down different foods.

Nutrients could never be absorbed into your blood without them; they are essential to life. Enzymes are found in foods and these highly sensitive protein molecules can be easily destroyed by chemical additives, by freezing and by cooking. If enzymes are not ingested daily via raw foods (pineapple, papaya, and apples are particularly good sources), proper digestion is impaired, leading to sickness and, I believe, hastening the aging process.

The process of digestion begins as soon as food enters your mouth. As you chew, breaking the food into smaller morsels, enzymes are secreted in your mouth. Your saliva moistens the particles until they are fully saturated. Rolled into a softened ball by your tongue, the food then passes down the alimentary canal into your stomach where other enzymes and hydrochloric acid,

160

the main gastric juice, are secreted, and the digestive process is furthered. For example, when you eat a starchy food such as bread or oatmeal, the enzyme ptyalin, which digests carbohydrates, is secreted in your mouth, changing these molecules into maltose, a sugar compound that will be further decomposed in your stomach.

The secretion of enzymes may be thought of as a clockwork operation. Each and every enzymatic agent is released according to the kind of food that has been eaten, whether it be an animal protein, starch, fruit or leafy green. Physiologist Emil Fischer offered what is probably the clearest explanation of the relationship between food and enzymes. Comparing this biochemical relationship to a lock and key, the food being the lock, the enzyme the key, he demonstrated that it takes a special key to open each different lock. If the key doesn't fit the lock exactly, then food will not be decomposed, and the process of digestion either will be retarded or not occur at all. The lock can only be opened, he explained, with the right enzymatic key.

Each enzyme acts in a highly specialized way: decomposing one and only one class of food. An enzyme that combines with a carbohydrate molecule will not react with a protein compound or a fat. The process is so specialized that an enzyme that acts on one kind of sugar molecule, such as maltose, will not decompose a related compound, such as lactose.

And because enzymes have such individualized functions, each stage of digestion requires different enzymes to break food down into its smallest assimilable parts. If, in a previous stage of digestion, a food has not been prepared for further digestion because the appropriate enzyme had been destroyed by a chemical additive or inhibited by the presence of a food substance of another class, the enzymes in the next stage of digestion will not be capable of performing their work.

Different classes of foods should, therefore, not be mixed at the same meal. Simultaneously eating a protein, for instance, and a starch impedes thorough digestion. I believe that when meat and potatoes, an all-American favorite, are chewed, ptyalin, the starch-reducing enzyme in the mouth, is inhibited by the acidic content of the meat. When the foods are passed into the stomach, gastric juices provide even more acidity, rapidly ending the digestive process. The food eventually passes from your body without giving you the full benefit of its nutrients.

In my opinion, combining any foods whose enzymes are not compatible has a similar effect on your digestive system. For instance, the acid content of a fruit such as an orange or an apple is sufficient to destroy the ptyalin of the saliva and impede the digestion of a starch such as bread or brown rice. Similarly, a fruit's acidity inhibits the gastric juices by destroying or stopping the secretion of pepsin, the enzyme that catalyzes the breakup of complex protein compounds into smaller substances in the stomach. Proteins and fruits should, therefore, never be combined. Since the high acidic level of fruit can also, I believe, impede the digestion of vegetables, these two types of food should be eaten at different meals.

Just as different sugar molecules cannot be broken down by the same enzymes, different proteins require specific gastric enzymes. In my opinion, these enzymes will conflict, neutralizing each other. Therefore, more than one kind of protein should not be eaten at the same meal. As you can see in the Time of Digestion Chart on pages 174–75, eggs are digested within a half-an-hour while meat can take up to three to four hours to be completely decomposed. Lamb goes through the process in one or two hours and veal or turkey take three hours. Eating eggs with fish, or cheese with chicken will release different enzymatic agents, thus preventing the proper reduction of each protein compound into less complex molecules. Therefore, my rule is to eat only one kind of protein at a meal.

Looking at the Food-Combination Chart on page 176, we see that protein and vegetables, or starch and vegetables can be eaten together. Fruits, as noted, should be eaten separately. Different fruits have varying pH values (acid/alkaline levels); an orange, for example, is highly acidic and a papaya more alkaline. Therefore, eat only one kind of fruit at a time. Many nutritionists believe that fruits can be mixed, for example, as in a fruit cup. I have found however, that the different acid/alkaline levels of different fruit definitely retard their digestion if they are eaten in combination.

As with all other aspects of the diet, work slowly into combining your foods properly. Don't build up inner pressure or feel stressed by this change in your diet. I have found that emotional stress actually causes the indiscriminate secretion of enzymes, which interferes with proper digestion, and results in the formation of toxicity.

When modifying your current diet to the proper food combinations, remember that different foods require different lengths of time to be broken down. There is no point in eating a properly combined meal if you are going to rush into eating a dessert or beverage before the entrée has been thoroughly digested. If you refer to the Time of Digestion Chart, you will see that vegetables such as asparagus, spinach, squash and carrots take one to two hours to be broken down in the stomach. Starches such as brown rice, buckwheat and oatmeal also require one to two hours. Animal proteins such as veal, lamb, chicken and liver take from one to three hours, while fish such as halibut, haddock and sole take two hours, and salmon three hours. Fruits, like vegetables, also require one to two hours to be digested. Note also that some of the more common American staples—bacon, french fried potatoes, cooked pork, American cheese, clams and rich dressings, sauces and gravies—are the most difficult foods to digest, requiring four to five hours for simplification into smaller compounds.

Ideally, you should wait for the full time required for the digestion of one food before eating a food of another class or drinking a liquid. However, if you are not accustomed to spacing your meals over a long period of time, or if your occupation restricts your lunch breaks, try to wait at least half-an-hour to forty-five minutes before having your next course. If you work in an office, I suggest that you take your fruit or beverage back to your desk, wait the prescribed amount of time, and then (if you are not under pressure or feeling tense), eat the fruit or dessert or drink the beverage.

The longer you allow your food to digest before additional eating or drinking, the more nutritional value you will receive.

If knowledgeable selection and the proper combination of foods are the first two fundamental steps in the art of eating, knowing *when* to eat is next in importance. Taste buds entice man into nourishing himself, and make eating a pleasurable experience. Eating, of course, sustains life, but, for many people, eating has been transformed from an essential act to an habitual indulgence.

The average American eats for many reasons—few of them the right ones. He eats as a means of social communication. Friends get together around a coffee table or at the bar and business is often conducted at the lunch table.

Food is also a wonderful palliative, often used to soothe one's depressions or restlessness. How many times has a snack of bread and butter, cookies, cake or an ice-cream sundae consoled you?

The majority of people eat at certain times because they have been conditioned. Whether it's nine in the morning or twelve noon, their stomachs and salivary glands, in a conditioned reflex, anticipate the coming morsels, and automatically begin to secrete their enzymes. When I had an office in New York City, I always knew it was noontime because my mouth would water and my stomach growl anticipating the food prepared at a dairy restaurant where I habitually lunched. It took me months to finally gain some control over these reactions and recondition myself so that I no longer "couldn't wait to eat."

There are also people whose bodies crave foods because of certain disorders, such as a person with hypoglycemia who, I believe, always hungers for sugar.

I am convinced that one should eat *only* when hungry. However, because most people are conditioned to eat according to a schedule or directed by body cravings, or (in most cases) by a desire to gratify their taste buds, they rarely experience true hunger. When the body requires food to empower it, the taste

164

buds are activated. This is the genuine physiological sign that food is needed. When that desire has been satisfied, the hunger ceases and the taste buds "shut off" so to speak. When the body is hungry again, it will again "tell you" to take some food by reactivating the taste buds.

In the past few years there have been many recommendations by nutritionists and scientists concerning the number of meals a person should eat during the day to sustain and nourish himself. The standard American diet is a hearty breakfast of juice, cereal, eggs, bacon and toast, followed by a sandwich or two and a fruit and beverage at lunch, ending the day with a four-course meal consisting of a salad, soup, meat and a pastry. Some nutritionists have said that the best diet is a solid breakfast, then a light lunch— a sandwich or a fruit—and then a solid three-course dinner at the end of the day. Others, including Russian scientists, have claimed that breaking heavy meals into four or five light snacks is less of a stress on the digestive system and provides the body with a constant supply of food. Then, there are those people who eat one meal a day—beginning at breakfast, and nibbling their way right through to dinner!

It's my opinion that when the body is in a healthy state, it requires only two meals a day. Provided the stomach has been shrunk to its normal size—most people's stomachs are four to five times normal size, which is a little larger than a fist—the body can comfortably perform on breakfast and dinner without weakening or suffering from nutritional deficiency. (This in fact was the diet of many early pioneers and farmers who settled this country.)

The word "breakfast" literally means what it says: to "break the fast." The day should begin as follows (this, of course, depends upon your blood type and current state of health): a glass of juice, a cup of cereal and a slice of toast or a boiled egg. For a high-protein breakfast you can include tofu, or substitute two eggs, soft cheese and tofu. The main meal should be at dinner, consisting of a salad, steamed vegetables, fish or meat or grain, depending upon your blood type.

Because many people find this regimen too strict for them, and for those patients undergoing a healing treatment requiring greater than average nourishment, I suggest the inclusion of a lunch meal, which can be a salad and bread, salad and cheese or eggs, or the main meat or grain meal, with a salad dinner.

But, I must repeat, the body will be perfectly satisfied with two meals a day. The long space between meals will enable the digestive system to rest and during this period the enzyme-secreting cells resupply the necessary enzymatic particles so that the next meal can be effectively digested. If one eats between meals, or has a heavy meal three times a day, long periods are required for digestion. Enzyme regeneration halts, the current supply of enzymatic particles is further depleted, and the present and future efficiency of the digestive system is greatly diminished. This, I feel sure, places a tremendous strain on the entire alimentary tract. It's like asking a marathon runner who has just crossed the finish line to run a few more miles.

A digestive system that receives adequate rest is able to digest a meal thoroughly. This will eliminate many disruptive gastric disorders, including dyspepsia, gastritis and flatulence.

An illustration of this is the case of one of my patients, a housewife in her forties who was a compulsive eater. She had an advanced case of hypoglycemia and began eating upon rising in the morning, consuming three hearty meals as well as numerous snacks of candy, pumpernickel laden with strawberry preserves, dried fruits and condensed milk with chocolate syrup. Her low-blood-sugar condition was accompanied by foul flatulence and chronic indigestion. Her sugar-rich snacks caused an increase in both her acidity and the activity of her gastric juices. I found that her acidity level was more than 25 percent above normal, and her enzyme activity had been raised by as much as 300 percent. During the treatment of her hypoglycemia, I put her on a low carbohydrate/high-protein diet, eliminating sugar-rich foods— chocolate, jams and jellies and dried fruit—and I temporarily reduced her intake of breads, grains and potatoes. Although she was a type B, her condition required an O regimen, recommending that she eat chicken twice and fish three times a week. Within a month, her embarrassing flatulence and acidic indigestion were largely reduced. As her low-blood-sugar condition came under control, her compulsive eating habits were relaxed and she found she could be satisfied with three meals a day, only occasionally reaching for a snack.

As Mr. Belvedere, the male nanny, emphasized, eating should be done in as quiet and relaxed an environment as possible. Excessive (or upsetting) talk at the table or quarrels while eating interfere with proper digestion. It's a one-way ticket to discomfort. Enzyme secretion is disrupted and an increased amount of air is swallowed with the meal. I have found that over 70 percent of all gastric-related disorders, such as distension, gastritis and flatulence are caused by upsetting conversation during meals.

While attending a conference for Naturopathic physicians in France, I noticed two French doctors having a heated row over lunch. Later in the day, I heard one complain of a bloated feeling, blaming it on the food. When it was his turn to address his fellow physicians, he was forced to end his speech abruptly when he developed a case of hiccups caused by the excessive air he had swallowed during lunch.

Eating when relaxed, and in silence, will help to safeguard the body from the undue ingestion of air, and will promote proper enzymatic secretion. Of course, when you're having dinner with friends or at a business luncheon, you have to talk. Your company would think there was something wrong with you if you remained mute. In my own home, I, myself, cannot always practice what I preach, for I am often lured into conversation at the dinner table by my youngest son, who is a real chatterbox. However, that little extra effort you can make to remain relaxed and quiet at a meal will go a long way in helping your body digest the food.

Here are a couple of suggestions for creating a peaceful ambience when you eat. Remove all potentially upsetting distractions such as television, the newspaper, or rock and roll music, which will undoubtedly unsettle your stomach with its pulsing rhythms. Not only does indiscriminate chatter disquiet your body, any obtrusive, upsetting sounds can also disturb the essential secretion of saliva and gastric juices.

If you are eating out, try to dine at a quiet, intimate type of restaurant. Avoid busy places where there's a lot of commotion—and never let your waiter rush you through your meal. Some restaurants in New York and other big cities are only interested in customer turnover and not the patron's comfort. Eat slowly, sit calmly for a short while after completing your meal, and then leave.

This brings us to Mr. Belvedere's second piece of advice, "Chew your food not fifty-five, or sixty-five but seventy-five times." This reminds me of an old saying my mother repeated to me when I was a boy: "After you've chewed your food forty times on one side of your mouth, chew it forty times on the other side." I don't know anybody who is going to count the number of times he chews his food! But, the importance of thorough mastication to digestion can't be emphasized enough. Digestive enzymes react only on the surface of food particles and not upon their interior, so that the rate of digestion is dependent upon the total surface area exposed to gastric and intestinal secretions. The more you chew your food, the greater the surface area becomes, and the effectiveness of digestion increases throughout the gastrointestinal tract. This, in turn, increases the ease with which food is passed from the stomach to the small intestines and other areas of the body, placing less of a strain on the digestive system.

Starches in particular, as they undergo digestion in the mouth, should be chewed and broken down as well as possible to facilitate the digestion of sugar molecules in the stomach.

People who love to eat but gulp their food down without properly chewing, also deprive themselves of one of the greatest pleasures: gratifying their taste buds. Only through thorough mastication is the full richness of the taste of food experienced. Many people don't realize that the taste of food is important in stimulating the gastric juices necessary for digestion. Taste buds are nerve endings, and when your body needs food, the taste buds become stimulated and entice you to eat. When food comes

168

into contact with these same taste buds, impulses are sent to the brain and then relayed to the stomach, so that the appropriate juices needed for the digestion of the food now being chewed may be secreted.

Because the secretion of gastric juices is initiated by the taste of food, chewing thoroughly and keeping the food in your mouth long enough to extract its full flavor helps prepare the stomach for proper digestion. This is also a very good reason why foods should be eaten as closely as possible to the plain and simple state in which they are found in nature. By disguising your foods with condiments, spices, and sauces, the true taste is hidden. The message from the brain to the stomach can thereby be confused, inhibiting the release of the proper digestive juices.

Chewing food well also expedites proper digestion because it warms the food and this accelerates the catalytic activities of the enzymes. Swallowing cold foods whole slows the digestive process by inhibiting the proper secretion of enzymes.

Lastly, proper mastication helps you to control the amount of food you eat. Overeating has become one of our most difficult and dangerous health problems. Millions of Americans are bloated and dyspeptic because of the way they stuff themselves. Overweight people have a mortality rate several times higher than people of normal weight in the same age groups. They are also more vulnerable to heart attacks, and their rate of diabetes and vascular disorders is much higher than that of persons of normal weight.

When you overeat, you literally become drunk with food. The blood in your body is immediately drawn to your stomach to help digest the meal, and lethargy and sleepiness ensue. This is a very common occurrence during holiday seasons when families get together to celebrate over huge dinners. In the course of the celebration, they usually forget about good nutrition and gorge themselves. Then they are too tired to carry on with the festivities, and before retiring usually have to take an antacid to settle their gurgling, distended bellies.

A patient of mine, who is an executive on Wall Street, told me that his colleagues all say, "If you want to get any work done, do it before lunch." Lunch for these businessmen is usually a large meal with cocktails and a few glasses of wine, which leads to a common midafternoon lethargy. My patient assured me that productivity is cut by nearly 50 percent after twelve o'clock.

Moreover, when you eat excessively, the walls of your stomach stretch like an inflated balloon. Although stomach muscles are elastic and were created to contract and expand, when they are grossly enlarged the cells of the abdominal walls undergo a tremendous strain, resulting, I have found, in an imbalance of the hydrochloric-acid level in the stomach and ulcers. One of my patients had violated his stomach so badly by overeating that he actually had perforations in his stomach walls.

You can avoid overeating by properly masticating food, because slow, meticulous chewing diminishes the sensation of hunger. When you eat rapidly and gulp your food without chewing, your taste buds will never be satisfied and you will continue to gorge yourself long after you've eaten all the food necessary for your nourishment.

Our eating habits have been conditioned from early childhood, and are a very strong part of our lives, so they must be slowly transformed and gradually replaced. Sometimes it takes twice as much effort to break a habit as it does to form one! When you are at the table, whether alone or with your family, become aware of the act of eating. Before you start to eat, think of what you are trying to accomplish. Let this thought sink in so that it is always there to guide you. Then proceed.

When you are at a table with food before you, think about its purpose: it is there to nourish you. (I tell my patients to remember, "Today's food is tomorrow's fuel.") Eating the wrong food, overeating, eating rapidly without masticating properly are impediments to proper digestion; if you do any of these things you are harming yourself.

Take your first mouthful of food and chew it slowly. While chewing, place your fork or spoon on your plate. This will help

170

prevent you from shoveling in one mouthful after another; and help you to create a slower rhythm of eating. This should be practiced at every meal, but if you fail to adopt this habit right away, don't feel pressured or upset. Remember, as long as the thought has been planted in your mind, it will return to you; and over a period of time, you will remind yourself to eat more slowly until eventually this will become your new habit.

During the meal, if you feel suddenly nervous or anxious, put down your fork or spoon, take a deep breath, relax, and then begin to eat again. (It is also a good idea to practice some form of deep breathing throughout the meal to release any knots or tension in your stomach muscles and thereby facilitate proper digestion.) If you must talk at a meal, avoid heated discussions or any negative conversation. Try not to complain or criticize, for doing so will only charge your emotions and disturb your digestive system. Try to talk about something pleasant or positive; about something good that happened to you today, or about a person's good qualities. Save your complaints and criticisms for after dinner. Often a person home from work has had to drive on busy highways or ride crowded buses or trains and is tired and grumpy. At the dinner table, there is talk about the argument with the boss, the inadequacies of the transportation system, or complaints about how unkempt the house or garden is: only negative feelings are vented. It's a rare individual who can come home after a hard day with cheerful and positive thoughts. But, be aware of your thoughts and, considering how they can affect your digestion, try to find a subject of conversation that is pleasant and relaxing.

During the meal, try also to maintain an awareness of your stomach. The object of eating is to provide you with nourishment, not to fill your belly like a Christmas stocking. Before you feel full or bloated, tell yourself that this is all the food you need for nourishment. Make an effort to reduce your amount of food because by doing this you will condition yourself to respond to your stomach instead of nervous hunger. Each day you will

171

actually find that you are eating a little less food. Slowly, your stomach will begin to shrink to its normal size and eventually smaller and fewer meals a day will satisfy your hunger.

Drinking with meals is another habit that disrupts the digestive system. Any liquid—and this means water, fruit and vegetable juices, soup, wine, beer and soda pop—dilutes the gastric juices, alters their acid/alkaline level and slows down digestion. In addition, any liquid that contains a potentially toxic substance, such as coffee, tea and cola (which have a high caffeine content), further retards digestion.

Most people drink something before or during a meal, and this habit may be difficult to break. But bear in mind reducing or eliminating your intake of liquids with meals can spare you a lot of digestive discomfort. If you are not experiencing such distress, refraining from drinking at meals will make it easier for your digestive system to work efficiently, help prevent future digestive disorders, and increase the nutritional values of your food.

If you wish to drink before a meal, have a glass of water (the least viscous fluid) fifteen minutes before you eat. It will pass through your stomach and intestines rapidly without interfering with the digestion of a meal. If you drink a fruit juice before breakfast, wait thirty to forty-five minutes before eating.

The amount of time to wait before drinking after meals is determined by the length of time it takes to digest certain foods. You should familiarize yourself with the Time of Digestion Chart and if, for example, you had broiled salmon for dinner, wait three hours before drinking anything. (In consulting the chart, always check for the food you have eaten that takes the *longest* amount of time to be digested.) Drinking liquids prematurely floods the stomach and dilutes hydrochloric acid at a crucial time, thus retarding digestion.

Liquids should never be drunk either hot or cold. Enzymatic agents are dependent upon the proper temperature and warm (or room) temperatures are most conducive to their actions. Taking a cold liquid or food such as ice cream after a meal reduces the enzymes' digestive powers. On the other hand, hot liquids raise the temperature of the mouth and stomach above normal internal temperature, which also interferes with proper digestion.

Other factors that inhibit the digestive process include: eating when fatigued, chilled or overheated, or when not hungry. Every day, people violate their digestive systems in many of these ways and then they spend their money to buy remedies to temporarily relieve their gastric disorders. All these disorders—flatulence, ulcers, distension, acidity and gastritis—could be avoided if the digestive system were allowed to work without interference on properly digested food.

In my opinion, any food not efficiently digested and absorbed by the body causes and supports the growth of undesirable bacteria. When such bacteria are present, flatulence, foul-smelling stool and halitosis quickly follow. A properly digested protein food is broken down into its component amino acids. When they are not properly digested, I believe that proteins decompose by bacterial infestation, and like food left too long in the cupboard or even in the refrigerator, they are broken down into a variety of nonusable substances, such as ptomaines, which are poison. In my opinion, a starch, which under normal digestive conditions is broken down into simple sugars, can ferment and be transformed into carbon dioxide, acetic acid and alcohol, also nonusable poisons, when it has not been properly decomposed.

When a body is overloaded with foods the digestive system does not function normally: proteins do not yield their amino acids, nor starches their sugars, nor fruits their vitamins. Instead of these substances, which are vital for rebuilding and nourishing the cells of the body, I have found that toxicity increases, fats become rancid in the stomach, intestines do not provide essential fatty acids and glycerol, and vitamins and minerals are not absorbed into the bloodstream.

Besides the many discomforts associated with bad eating habits, interference with the digestive process also impairs clarity of thought and diminishes your ability to reason and create. My studies have shown that toxicity has a wearing and draining effect on all the body's systems—and this is not something that can be instantly remedied by an Alka-Seltzer or a Bromo.

Only if you develop the right eating habits can your body make proper use of the foods that you have now so diligently begun to choose. Moreover, good eating habits will help you relieve some of the most common gastric disorders that afflict people worldwide.

My studies have shown these relationships between various foods and the time required for their digestion.

TIME OF DIGESTION

Five Minutes to Digest
White of the egg; yolk of the egg; bouillon, honey, butter and olive oil

One Hour to Digest
Roasted almonds, asparagus, apples (sweet and ripe), arrowroot, cooked barley, lean beef, young beets, cantaloupe, chicken broth, green corn, cornmeal, cream, dates, figs, grapefruit, whole-wheat flour, lamb, lettuce, milk, Irish moss (carrageen), olives, onions, oranges, oysters, peaches, prunes, plums, peas, baked potatoes, raisins, brown rice, spinach, strawberries, squash, watermelon

Two Hours to Digest
Artichokes, beans, buckwheat, capon, chicken, carrots, codfish, cream cheese, herring, haddock, halibut, lentils, filberts (hazelnuts), oatmeal, parsnips, new potatoes, rye, sole, salsify, tomatoes, trout, turkey and veal

Three Hours to Digest

Old beets, cauliflower, cabbage, canned corn, flounder, boiled ham, salted herring, liver, lobster, pecan nuts, hickory nuts, dried peas, sweet potatoes, salmon, cooked spinach, venison

Four Hours to Digest

Bacon, brown bread, old beans, crabs, duck, doughnuts, lard, cooked meats, recooked meats, pork, fried oysters, fried onions, peanuts, walnuts, fried potatoes, old turnips

Five Hours to Digest

Whole barley, barley bread, American cheese, clams, fried ham, oily nuts, cooked pork, pastries, pie crusts, shrimp, chopped meat, fruit puddings, fruitcakes, rich sauces, dressings and gravies

FOOD-COMBINATION CHART

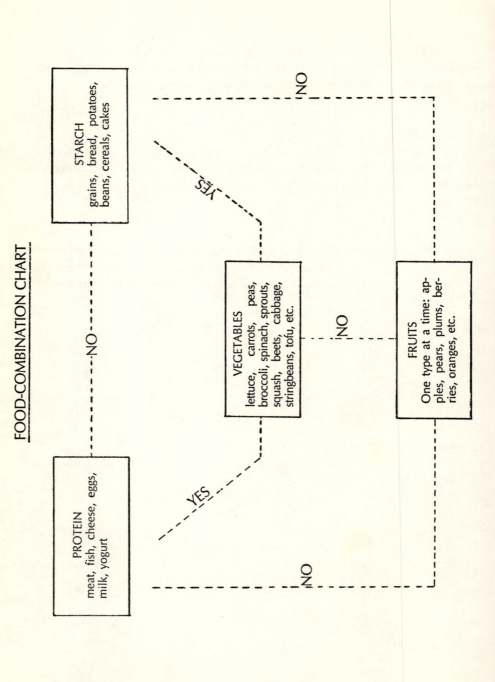

STARCH
grains, bread, potatoes, beans, cereals, cakes

PROTEIN
meat, fish, cheese, eggs, milk, yogurt

VEGETABLES
lettuce, carrots, peas, broccoli, spinach, sprouts, squash, beets, cabbage, stringbeans, tofu, etc.

FRUITS
One type at a time: apples, pears, plums, berries, oranges, etc.

NO

NO

YES

YES

NO

NO

10

Cleansing the Body

Throughout this book I've made many suggestions on what and how you should eat. I've recommended foods that will benefit your individual body, explained the proper way of eating, and recommended various basic techniques with which you can nourish and care for yourself.

However, equally important in the treatment of a run-down or diseased body, and fundamental to my health care program, is the elimination of substances I have found to be toxic, such as uric acid, mucus and acidity that have accumulated in your body's tissues and organs.

I am convinced that the retention of wastes is, without a doubt, one of the main factors contributing to the deterioration of body strength as well as the cause of many common illnesses such as arthritis, colitis, migraine headaches and heart attacks.

If we look at what happens to food when it enters the body, we can see that it is chewed in the mouth where it is prepared for digestion, then passed down the alimentary canal into the stomach, where it is broken down into assimilable substances, then funneled into the small intestines, where nutrients are absorbed for distribution around the body. Also produced during

177

these biochemic processes are unassimilable waste products which are normally passed to the large intestine (the colon) and excreted from the body.

However, because of the poor quality of food that most people eat and their improper eating habits, many have weakened and inefficient digestive and elimination systems. Consequently, food is not thoroughly digested nor waste products completely evacuated. The result I have found is clogging of the colon with acids, mucus, gas and hardened stool, leading to a toxic contamination of the entire system.

An examination of the structure of the colon shows that, unlike a tube or a pipe, its inner core is molded into arcs, or pockets. In a clean, healthy colon these "pockets" absorb toxic substances and help eliminate them from the body as well as assimilating the remaining nutrients not absorbed in the small intestines.

It has been estimated that roughly 85 percent of the assimilation of nutrients occurs in the twenty-eight feet of the small intestines. Nature, being frugal, wanted man to receive the maximum benefit from his food, and so provided him with an additional five to six feet of intestinal muscle, the colon. This division of the large intestine completes the assimilation of the remaining 15 percent of digested nutrients and helps to eliminate wastes.

In my opinion the colon in most people is caked with toxic matter, so that the remaining nutrients cannot be fully absorbed by the blood. I believe that not only is the body thereby deprived of its full nourishment, but that, during the assimilation of food in the colon, small amounts of poisonous wastes lining this organ are sucked into the blood and circulated around the body.

Furthermore, I believe that when the body is hungry and the stomach or small intestines lack food to absorb, the colon automatically responds and tries to supply the nutrients—but instead of nourishing the body's hungry cells with vital nutrients, it sends them toxic wastes.

The colon can really be thought of as a sewer system. And, I have found that if that system is clogged with waste matter, the evacuation of unassimilable toxic materials will be prevented and, like any drainpipe, back up so that the effluent will flow through other available openings. In the twelfth century, the Hebrew philosopher/physician Maimonides described how this can affect one: "If the body does not eliminate properly, first the mind becomes tense and nervous, and then the body becomes diseased."

Besides giving man's body an opportunity to make use of a great percentage of the nutrients it ingests, Nature also gave him a protective filtration system to remove any undesirable substances that seep into the bloodstream. Here's a brief description of how it works.

As blood passes through the kidneys, uric acids and other morbid matter are filtered out. Whatever wastes are not removed by the kidneys will continue to circulate in the blood and will be dealt with by other organs, such as the lungs. If organs, such as the kidneys, are constantly forced to filter out a large supply of wastes, they will falter and eventually break down, like any machine that is overworked. Then such disorders as kidney stones and gouty arthritis can develop. In addition, if the kidneys can no longer cope with the wastes, the poisons will automatically spill over into the bladder, which is unequipped to perform the necessary filtration. I believe that in a woman, this can imbalance the level of cleansing flora (friendly bacteria) in the uterus and cause vaginal discharge and cystitis. In a man, malfunctioning kidneys can inflame his prostate gland.

When the blood passes through the lungs for purification, I believe that a fairly high level of toxicity will irritate the sensitive mucus membranes, resulting in the production of catarrh in the respiratory system. Disorders such as chest congestion, asthma or, in my opinion, many kinds of allergies, such as hay fever, can then occur.

The liver is another organ busy working to keep the blood pure and healthy. One of the most important activities of the liver, the largest gland of the body, is to manufacture bile. (Bile is stored by the gallbladder and helps to emulsify fats, among other essential functions.) The liver also tries to break down waste products into simpler compounds more easily filtered by the kidneys. If the liver, which I believe to be the main natural defense against all forms of toxicity, can no longer render toxic wastes harmless (especially certain toxic chemicals like the nitrogenous fertilizers that often seep into water supplies), I am sure that these toxins will be absorbed by the cells and destroy the vital enzymes controlling the energy-respiratory mechanism, resulting in a severe reduction of cell oxidation. When a fundamental biological action such as normal cell respiration is inhibited, the entire body loses its vital strength and becomes susceptible to many serious diseases.

One other important organ of elimination is the skin. Wastes not filtered out from the blood will try to seep through the skin's pores, in my opinion. Acids will be discharged from the body as it perspires. Clear or gummy fluids, or pus, may be discharged through the skin, causing, in my opinion, such skin problems as eczema, psoriasis, boils or shingles. The mucous membranes in the nose will manufacture catarrh, and the eyes may exude pus or develop styes. The ears can discharge a dark waxy substance, and the mouth may develop canker sores.

The body makes every effort, using all its internal and external equipment, to keep itself pure and clean. It is obvious that whatever nourishment enters the body must be digested and used efficiently, while the waste products must be completely discharged. If they are not, and the elimination system can no longer do its work effectively, disease can ensue.

The question now arises, "How can I help my digestive and elimination systems work efficiently?" First, having bowel movements every day will prevent the buildup of caked waste matter in the colon, and I am convinced that this will prevent the absorption of toxic materials by the blood. I have found that people have very peculiar notions about what a regular bowel movement is. Some think that if they eliminate once a day it's sufficient. Others believe once every two days is normal. I've had patients who thought moving their bowels once a week was okay.

180

A comparison of a healthy colon with the colon of a teenage girl who eliminated once a week revealed that her transverse section and descending colon were swollen and sagging. The patient with this abnormality suffered extreme lethargy, moodiness, antisocial behavior and an inability to concentrate in school. I discovered that her improper elimination habits had caused her body to retain so much toxicity that her cells were being devitalized by the poisons: consequently she had no pep, had become grumpy and was not able to be mentally focused and alert. I recommended a special vegetarian diet and certain herbal laxatives for this girl. Within a week, her entire attitude toward people and school had been reversed.

I believe that, ideally, wastes should be eliminated from the body at least three times a day. If you don't eliminate with this regularity, I suggest that you try conditioning yourself to this habit by simply going to the toilet after each meal. The bowels are muscles and they can be trained. Just sit on the toilet and relax. Don't force yourself because this can distend your hemorrhoidal vein and cause hemorrhoids. Few people eliminate the first few times, but soon, you will find that your bowels will respond.

Other ways you can promote proper bowel movements are by: eating salads two to three times a day; eating such fruits as prunes or plums; drinking the juice of half a lemon in warm water followed by two glasses of cool water; adding bran to your cereal; or drinking an herbal tea composed of fern, caraway seeds, chamomile and golden seal.

Herbal laxatives, which are available at health stores, and enemas (used only for brief periods of time primarily when you are constipated) can also safely aid proper elimination.

However, the most common worldwide method of "cleansing" the body is the fast. Since ancient times, people have fasted both to recover their health and to enhance their spiritual awareness. I personally have seen countless cases of patients suffering severe skin eruptions, goiter, backaches, stiff and swollen joints recover a tremendous amount of their lost health by fasting.

One of the most striking cases of my career was that of an old woman I treated when I worked in Norway. She was a frail woman in her sixties, who possessed an unusual inner strength. She had an advanced case of rheumatoid arthritis: her fingers and toes were bent at the joints and her body was severely hunched. I worked with this woman for a year, putting her on a series of water and fruit fasts (she required fruit for nourishment because her body was very weak). Sometimes she fasted for several days, sometimes for nearly a week. After a year of alternating between a special diet and fasting, her skeletal system had recovered such a degree of flexibility that many of her fingers and toes straightened out and regained their mobility. She could also now stand erect.

Fasting is a highly controversial topic among nutritionists. Some believe that although it helps to detoxify, a lack of proper nourishment can weaken the body and make it prone to illness. Others believe that it is a fundamental therapy. I strongly believe that fasting is one of the best ways to help cleanse the body: but only at the right time and under certain circumstances. When done improperly or at the wrong time, fasting has serious drawbacks.

If a patient is ill, I do not advise fasting. These are my reasons. I believe that waste lodges in the colon's "pockets" in the following way: gas is trapped and forced to the bottom of the "pocket" where it is covered by a layer of mucus, then a layer of acids, coated at the cusp by a resinous substance. During a fast, when the body hungers, it responds, as I explained previously, by first "asking" the stomach and small intestines for food; then, finding no nutrients in those two organs, the colon is, so to speak, alerted to supply the body with food. However, if the colon is lined with poisonous wastes, these substances will be circulated throughout the body.

In my experience, although a fast can help purify many of the body's tissues and organs by breaking up and discharging large amounts of toxic deposits (thereby remedying chronic symptoms

182

and illnesses), the reabsorption of waste matter secreted from the colon can cause other, though different, illnesses in the future.

For example, a top fashion model, who insisted on fasting for two weeks against my advice, experienced what I knew to be a release of toxicity into her body resulting in serious facial blemishes. She then sought surgery as a quick remedy, and had the blemishes peeled away and even new skin grafted onto her face.

Another argument against fasting is that the reduction in carbohydrate intake can cause abnormal body chemistry. Because the main fuel of the brain is glucose (blood sugar), a severe reduction of carbohydrates can, I have found, cause a loss of emotion control, including such reactions as anxiety, depression, spontaneous weeping, violent outbursts and an intense mistrust of people.

Despite these considerations, I believe fasting can be highly beneficial to you, but only after you have been on the diet for at least six months. Fasting should never be attempted if you are still weak or ill. (If you are uncertain about your state of health consult your doctor.) If you have been on one of my diets, and have been taking vitamins and eliminating regularly, it is probable that your body is strong and has already discharged a lot of toxicity. At this point, fasting can help eliminate many of the remaining wastes in your body, including any embedded matter in your colon. The type of fast that I recommend is a three-day grapefruit-juice fast. It should be conducted as follows.

First, create a peaceful environment for yourself. Restrict all external influences that may upset you. Avoid reading newspapers or watching TV because they tire or excite you. Refrain from any strenuous activity because your body will not have the nutrients necessary for excessive expenditure of energy.

Upon awakening the first morning, take time to calm yourself. Meditate, take a lukewarm bath, or sit quietly to prepare for the day. When you feel quiet and relaxed, drink a glass of freshly squeezed, unsweetened grapefruit juice diluted with water (half-juice, half-water). Throughout the day, drink fifteen more glasses of diluted grapefruit juice for nourishment, and to help purify your body.

Before going to bed, drink a mixture of lemon juice and olive oil (one squeezed lemon to an equal part olive oil). This will act as a mild laxative. Repeat this program for three days in all.

During the first day, you will probably experience fatigue and have a great desire to eat. Rest or nap during the day. On the second day, you may be overcome by a great feeling of exhaustion. You may also have a bad taste in your mouth, body odor and some minor skin irritations. These are common reactions caused, in my experience, by the release of toxins from your body. On the third day, you should experience a tremendous surge of energy and a feeling of unusual body lightness.

When you are coming off the fast on the fourth day, eat only the most laxative of foods—steamed or raw vegetables. Avoid breads and grains, meats and cheese. Let your body continue to eliminate freely. Heavy foods can be difficult to digest because your digestive system has been inoperative for three days. On the fourth night, drink the lemon juice and olive oil mixture again to help discharge any remaining wastes.

If your life-style prohibits a three-day fast, try a one-day fast, drinking fifteen glasses of grapefruit and taking lemon juice and olive oil before retiring.

During your fast, examine your stool. Some substances that you might see are white strands of mucus, or green balls (which in my experience indicate a bilious nature), or hard coral-like matter, which in my opinion is old stool that may have been encrusted in your colon for as long as fifteen to twenty years.

Become aware of temperature changes, odors, and gas when you eliminate. I have found that a foul smell indicates putrefaction and a release of wastes; gas suggests that you are eating too quickly and swallowing air, or that you are combining your foods improperly; and a sudden rush of heat from your rectum means that you are passing acids.

In my experience, many people have greatly improved their health through the purification of their bodies. Athletes have gained more energy, students have increased their attention span and ability to learn and people with nervous conditions have become calmer. One of my patients who was helped by just one three-day fast was a writer who needed a nap twice a day. When I first treated him, I thought his tiredness was due to his hypoglycemic condition. However, after following a low-carbohydrate/high-protein diet for eight months, this patient's disorder was healed and yet he was still tired and enervated. Had I not reexamined him I might have decided that it was "writer's block"; perhaps a means of escaping his work. However, after I had examined his eyes, I realized that his body was still very toxic. I recommended that he fast and he did. The next time I saw him he was a different man: his face was more animated, the circles under his eyes were gone; his body radiated a new-found vitality, and he no longer needed his daily naps!

Another of my cases was that of a woman in her forties involved in the fashion world, who came to me after experimenting with many different cosmetics. She had already had one facelift and was in despair because her skin was wrinkling. I told her that no beauty treatments, makeup, or facelifts could halt the aging process or improve the quality of her skin. However, I also told her that her complexion could become clearer, regaining a youthful texture, if her body was purified by fasting. She took the challenge. After she had fasted several times over a six-month period, she reported triumphantly that people were amazed at how young she looked. Furthermore, her career took an upswing—she was hired by a cosmetic company to endorse their product!

I believe that only by purifying yourself of accumulated toxic matter can you get the full value from your diet and recover maximum health.

In the next chapter, I will tell you about many other therapies, including herbal teas and baths, water and clay treatments and the use of color, that can also aid in cleansing your body to recharge it with youthful vigor.

11

Home Therapies

It is not enough for man to beg his Creator for health and a long life: he should also use his intelligence to discover and bring to light treasures graciously hidden by God in Nature as a means of healing the ills of this human life.

—Sebastian Kneipp

At the beginning of this book I told you that Naturopathy was a broad art and science, incorporating many therapies. Now, I will try to explain how some of these treatments, including herbal teas and applications, water, clay, and the use of color can hasten the purification of the body and help to heal certain common illnesses.

First, however, I must reemphasize how important it is to take wise measures to guard your body against disease and prevent illness. Remember, the body harbors small amounts of just about every strain of bacteria in existence. Given the right condition—weakened resistance—the bacteria will multiply and other pathogens can invade your body and cause infection. A nourished body has a high resistance to disease, and even though your friends or family may contract colds or the flu, your natural defenses will usually be strong enough to insure your continued good health.

In addition, it is important that your body excrete its wastes regularly and efficiently. Even though it is properly nourished, the body that retains waste will not be functioning properly and this will make it prone to bacterial or other infestation.

To repeat: My fundamental health program is directed toward nourishing your body and keeping it free of toxic materials.

Many therapies used by Naturopaths, such as vitamins, are supplementary healing aids. Nevertheless, they can play an important role in remedying a disorder. Herbs, for instance, which are plants and not drugs, heal, like other foods, through their nutritive properties. For example, burdock root feeds the capillaries in the scalp, thus stimulating the circulation of blood to the hair roots, which helps maintain the health of the hair. Another herb, black currant leaves, soothes the mucous membranes in the respiratory tract and alleviates nasal congestion. Water and clay may help heal infected tissues or organs by drawing out toxicity. I have found that by applying compresses (such as a towel soaked in cold water) to the stomach, and by taking certain kinds of baths, such as a tepid footbath, one can help decrease infection or congestion and relieve headaches and head colds.

COLOR THERAPY

My experience has shown that various colors heal the body through vibratory effects. For instance, yellow has a healing effect on the pancreas, whereas blue tranquilizes the central nervous system.

All color therapy treatments should be performed with a fifteen-watt bulb. Bulbs in the appropriate colors may be purchased at hardware and lighting-supply stores. Screw the colored bulb into any lamp (the small, inexpensive lamps with flexible stems are good for this purpose) and make sure the colored light is at least three feet away from the body. Use the appropriate color therapy for fifteen to twenty minutes. The effect of therapy will be enhanced further if you wear the appropriate color as much as possible and try to use it in your surroundings. (See color recommendations for the different blood types in chapter 4.)

COLOR THERAPY CHART

RED—Red radiates heat and stimulates the nervous system and metabolic functions. The red frequency raises body temperature, quickens the reaction of the heart and increases circulation, especially of arterial blood, which is drawn to the surface of the skin.

Skin and glands are activated by red light; it is also relieving to congested vital organs. Red can be harmful in inflammatory conditions and extended use can irritate the cerebrospinal and sympathetic nervous systems. It should not be used extensively on the head and is not recommended for stout or heavy people.

ORANGE—Orange has a "freeing" action upon bodily and mental functions. It works very effectively on the spleen, and through its active rays, the essences of all foods are assimilated, classified and distributed throughout the body. Orange rays assert tremendous influence on the respiratory system and are highly beneficial in healing any disorder of the lungs, esophagus, trachea or larynx, especially any asthmatic-related illness. Psychologically, the orange rays help one to tolerate others, and at the same time strengthen the will. It is the recommended color for psychosomatic symptomatology.

YELLOW—Next to white light, yellow gives off maximum luminosity. Its action stimulates the liver and intestines, and it is therefore the purifier of the entire system, particularly the skin. Yellow is a "mental" ray, with a stimulating effect on the intellectual faculties, activating the logical and reasoning powers of the mind. It aids in self-control by inspiring the higher faculties. It is also a color which brings one to a harmonious attitude toward life by providing balance and optimism. The use of yellow is recommended in cases of nervous exhaustion, especially when there are skin troubles, indigestion and related constipation, and liver trouble. Piles are also dramatically eliminated by the use of this color.

GREEN—Green is the color of Nature, balance, peace, and harmony. It controls the cardiovascular system and strongly influences the heart and blood pressure. A green environment will soothe the nerves. Its absence can promote irritability and hyperactivity. Green can be used to alleviate headaches, colds and the flu. Psychologically, green will bring one a feeling of renewal.

BLUE—Blue has a restricting action on body functions, slowing them down so that the body can combat infectious diseases or fevers. Blue can be used to help alleviate such diverse ailments as throat troubles, spasms, stings, shock, insomnia, headaches, itching and children's ailments such as measles and mumps. It is considered a great antiseptic, and palpitations, diarrhea, jaundice and colic are all helped by blue frequencies. Focused on the throat for periods of one-half hour, blue may help cure goiter. It is also effective in the treatment of gumboils and abscesses. Psychologically, blue can bring peace and quiet to the mind, particularly for those in overexcited states, such as hysteria.

INDIGO—Indigo is the color to use for mucus elimination. Mucus, fevers, whooping cough and pneumonia all warrant the use of this color. Psychologically, indigo soothes patients suffering from hallucinations, delusions, melancholia, hypochondria, hysteria, epilepsy, senile dementia and sexual overexcitement.

VIOLET—Violet is the color of all conscious energy. It acts in a soothing and tranquilizing manner on a frayed nervous system. However, its usefulness is mainly restricted to those people who are nervous or highly strung by nature. Violet light can be used for all mental and nervous disorders, as well as for rheumatism, concussions, kidney and bladder diseases, inflammatory diseases, and neuralgia.

SUPPLEMENTARY NATUROPATHIC REMEDIES

There are many other supplementary remedies that have been used by Naturopaths for hundreds of years. Let me give you an example from my own practice. A medical doctor, who is a patient of mine, was vacationing in Paris when he began to have terrible pains in his inner ear. He could easily have consulted a local medical doctor and received complementary treatment, but because I had helped to heal his case of colitis, he telephoned me to find out what treatment I would recommend. After he had described his condition, I suggested that he apply a baked potato to his ear three times a day until the pain abated. There was a moment of silence. Then, he very diplomatically told me that, while he respected my abilities, he felt that the treatment was a little far-fetched for him. I told him that I understood his reaction, but that it would work nevertheless. I reminded him that one of the quickest ways to cure frostbite is to apply snow to the frozen area and that this treatment (long used by the common people) is an example of one of the main principles of Natural Healing: "like cures like." I assured him the potato had certain properties that would draw the infection out and bring him relief. Reluctantly, he agreed to try it. Two days later he called me and though he was still in pain, I could sense his enjoyment in telling me that my treatment didn't work. I suggested that he heat some olive oil and pour a drop or two into his ear before again applying the baked potato. He was reluctant, but he seemed intrigued enough to try it. The following morning he called again, and putting professional pride aside, he thanked me for the cure! As you will read, there are other "far-fetched," but, I believe, reliable remedies.

In certain cases, when a disorder is deep-seated, or the impaired organ or system has not been diagnosed, the application of these remedies may not be totally effective; and if misused they can have an adverse effect on the body. If you are working with color therapy, and for example, you apply a red ray to stimulate your circulation while your body is in a state of nervous tension, a condition that calls for a yellow or blue light which can calm and soothe you, your nervous system could become overexcited, and your condition worsen. A careful analysis of your symptoms should help you choose the treatment required.

Lastly, the following recommendations do *not* represent a comprehensive guide to healing. Herbs alone would require a full book. My intention here is simply to give you a variety of suggestions that I have found valuable in healing some of the more common disorders.

ARTHRITIS This common condition suffered by people of all ages is, I believe, generally caused by an accumulation of uric acid and toxic matter in the body. In most cases, an excessive quantity of meat and dairy products has been consumed and their toxic by-products improperly evacuated. If you have arthritis, no matter what blood type you are, avoid all heavy meats and dairy products. If you are an A or AB, follow your regimen at level four in the rating charts. B's should enter at level three or four, eating fish twice a week. O's should start at level three, but temporarily avoid meat and dairy products, eating fish three times a week for protein.

All blood types should increase their intake of water from eight to ten to twelve glasses a day to help flush toxicities from the

192

kidneys and the bloodstream. Vegetables should be your main source of food in order to loosen your bowels for proper elimination. Exercise is also important, for it will help burn off circulating wastes.

If the arthritis is in the extremities of your body (hands and feet), soak those areas in rosemary tea. Steep a handful of rosemary in a pint of hot water, cool, then immerse the painful area into the tea. Do this several times a day to help relieve aches or stiffness. I believe that increasing your intake of calcium will promote flexibility in your joints and reduce the aches. If you are a type O or B, double your dosage of dolomite or bonemeal; types A and AB should increase their calcium lactate.

When arthritis is not localized in the extremities, take rosemary baths. Place a handful of herbs in a handkerchief and tie the ends to make a sack or sachet. Immerse it in the tub while the water is running and remain in the bath from ten to fifteen minutes. Do this two or three times a day, or as required. (Some herbs stain porcelain, so try to clean your bathtub immediately after bathing.)

Epsom salt baths can also be taken to draw out toxic wastes from the body. Add several tablespoons of the salt to a warm bath and allow it to dissolve before getting in. Continue running the water as you bathe, because a concentrated solution of Epsom salt has an extremely "drawing" (hypotonic) effect on the body. If you are a type A, or are older than forty, do not remain in the water for more than five to ten minutes because the solution will be particularly draining to you. It is also advisable to have someone help you get out of the bath, as you may feel faint and weak. Take Epsom salt baths in the evening and retire directly afterward.

To help ease local pains, you can massage the area with a gentle kneading action, or apply a clay poultice. (A poultice is an application of a wet cloth with an herb or clay. It helps to draw the toxicity from an inflaming or aching area and can be highly effective in soothing arthritic pains.) To make a poultice, put several tablespoons of white or yellow clay in a cup of water, and stir until a paste is formed. (Louvis Company No. 3 is a high-quality clay that I usually recommend; it is available at some health stores. However, if this is unavailable, any white French clay usually available at health stores will be suitable.) Place the mixture in a muslin cloth, apply to the aching area and secure it to your body by wrapping a warm wet towel around it. In cases of severe pain, you may wear the poultice overnight. Otherwise, apply for fifteen to twenty minutes, or as often as required.

Shining a blue or green light directly on the inflamed area for fifteen minutes every day will also help alleviate the pain and heal the condition.

In order to help cleanse your body, drink horsetail tea twice a day. If you are a type O or B, drink strong brews of the tea. A's and AB's should drink weak infusions because it can irritate their stomachs, possibly causing cramps or nausea. Strawberry-leaf tea may also be drunk twice a day by all blood types to help purify the blood.

These treatments may also be used in such related disorders as rheumatism, gout or bursitis.

ASTHMA—Dietary alterations for asthma are similar to those recommended for arthritis (see Arthritis).

To relieve acute attacks, create a steambath in your bathroom. Close the door, run hot water from your shower and inhale the vaporized air for fifteen minutes. This will help break up congestion and relieve coughing and wheezing.

Increasing your Vitamin A and C intake according to your blood type will help both to raise your body's resistance and heal the mucous membranes in your respiratory system. Focusing a blue or green light on your chest for fifteen minutes once or twice a day will also help to heal the mucous membranes. Hayseed flower baths, which will draw mucus and impurities from your body, should be taken twice a day. (If hayseed is unavailable, a clay or cold-water poultice may be applied to your chest to break up the congestion and improve breathing.)

To soothe and help heal your bronchial tracts, drink a brew of slippery-elm tea three times a day. Golden seal tea may also be drunk several times a day to assist in tissue repair.

INFLUENZA "The Flu"—It's my opinion that the flu only strikes those people whose resistance has been dissipated. Proper diet and elimination, and not overworking or stressing yourself during the cold winter months when the flu is most prevalent should be adequate protection against it.

However, if you do contract the flu, modify your diet by reducing your intake of meat, dairy products, and grains. Drink plenty of water and increase your consumption of citrus fruits and fruit juices. Proper elimination is important during the illness to help evacuate wastes.

To help disperse head congestion, take a fifteen-to-twenty-minute mustard footbath three times a day. Soaking your feet in a solution of one tablespoon of dried mustard in a basin of warm water will draw your blood down from your head and help break up congestion. A red light focused on your feet for fifteen minutes will have a similar effect.

Increase your Vitamin C intake according to your blood type and drink rose-hip tea (which has a high concentration of ascorbic acid) throughout the day to raise your body's resistance and strengthen your respiratory system. Golden seal tea can also be drunk twice a day or, as required, to help heal your mucous membranes and reduce your catarrhal condition.

FEVER—In my opinion, a fever is a general sign that your body is retaining toxic substances and is fighting to burn them off. This battle is what actually raises your body temperature. Resting in bed, staying warm and restricting your diet to steamed vegetables and citrus fruits are all vital in helping your body to discharge the foreign matter and thus lower your temperature.

Drinking golden seal tea three times a day will be beneficial to your mucous membranes. Rose-hip tea twice a day will be soothing to your lungs, and dandelion tea twice a day will stimulate your kidneys and flush acids from your body. In addition, water should be drunk throughout the day to replace the body fluids sweated off as your body eliminates the toxicity.

SORE THROATS—One of the most effective remedies I have found for a sore throat is to parboil a quarter of a cabbage, place it in a linen cloth and wrap it around your throat for half-an-hour. If you repeat this treatment several times a day (replacing the original cabbage with fresh pieces), it will reduce the inflammation by drawing out the toxins. Comfrey or hayseed-flower tea compresses, which are also very effective in reducing inflammations and soreness, may be applied to the throat two or three times a day. In addition, gargle five times a day with water and vinegar (white or apple-cider). Focusing a green light on your throat for fifteen minutes will also be beneficial.

Increasing your water intake will help flush impurities from your blood, and doubling your daily dosage of Vitamin C (according to your blood type) will increase your body's vitality and resistance, and help to heal inflamed tissues.

HERPES—These small infectious sores are caused by a virus and have been associated with nervous disorders. To prevent the proliferation and continuation of this condition, I believe that the body must be cleansed of waste matter.

I recommend a daily enema while the sores persist, and if the body is healthy and strong, a three-day fast. In addition, vitamin B_{12}, a B-complex formula and pantothenic acid should be increased (according to your blood type) to reduce the stress on your body. Dandelion or horsetail tea should be drunk three times a day to help cleanse the kidneys, and a green light should be focused on the kidney areas for fifteen minutes a day. Oatmeal packs (a handful of soaked rolled oats wrapped in linen cloth) or an oatmeal paste should be applied onto the infected areas three times a day to help dry up the sores.

The biochemic remedy is Kali. Phos., which is a nerve nutrient. For mild cases it should be taken twice a day; for more serious conditions take four times a day.

As herpes infections are, in my experience, often caused by a nervous condition, the real cure for this persistent skin disorder is the development of the right mental attitudes. Reflect quietly until you become aware of the cause of your emotional disturbance. This is a vital part of removing the problem. If not resolved, herpes sores will continue to spread, or will be temporarily healed only to return at a future time.

A boy of about five was brought to me after many fruitless attempts to cure this disorder by cauterizing (burning) the eruptions. He was a brave little fellow and apparently had undergone the treatments stoically, never wincing or complaining of the pain. During an interview with his mother, I discovered that his parents were divorced and that he rarely saw his father. When I asked him what he wanted more than anything else he quickly replied, "To play with my daddy." This was my clue. I suggested to his mother that we hold off beginning treatment, and that she make every effort to have the boy spend more time with her former husband. She arranged this. When she brought the boy back to me in three months he was much improved. Although his sores were not completely healed, many had receded and there were no new ones.

<u>SORE, INFLAMED EYES, OR CONJUNCTIVITIS</u>—Soak a handful of chamomile tea in a cup of hot water. Let cool, then soak your eye(s) in an eyecup of the solution for five to ten minutes, three times a day. For severe cases, bathe the eyes five to ten times a day. An infusion of eyebright or golden seal in water is also highly effective for inflammations of the eye (conjunctivitis).

BODY RASHES—Rashes of all types, including eczema, psoriasis and less severe eruptions such as boils or acne, are, I am sure, caused by the body's inability to discharge wastes through the normal exits of elimination—the bowels, lungs and kidneys. Since the toxicities are then excreted through the skin, the sensitive epidermal layer is irritated and rashes occur.

First, the body must be cleansed. To cleanse the kidneys and purify the blood, drink twelve glasses of water a day. Such fruits as grapefruits, peaches and watermelons should be eaten several times a day for they are good blood-purifiers. Drink dandelion tea twice a day to help cleanse the kidneys, and red-clover tea once a day to purify the blood. All spicy foods should be eliminated. Dairy products and grain intake should be reduced because these foods cause catarrh and increase the body's acidity by clogging the elimination system and irritating the kidneys.

Applying cold-water compresses over the kidneys is a highly effective method of drawing toxic wastes from the body. For a mild case, lie on your stomach and place the compress over your kidneys for fifteen minutes before retiring. For severe cases, secure the compress to your body by wrapping a towel or linen cloth around your waist and pinning it so that you can sleep with it in place overnight.

To help soothe irritated skin and stop itching, take oatmeal baths two to three times a day, or as needed. Place a handful of oatmeal in two handkerchiefs tied to make a bag and immerse this in warm water. The "milk" of the oatmeal will coat your rashes and stop the itching almost instantly. Local applications of a soaked oatmeal bag can also be held to the inflamed area.

DOUCHES—I believe that the menstrual period should always be followed by a douche to wash out any lingering wastes, such as blood clots, from the uterus. Both the common vinegar-and-water and the golden seal douches are recommended. To make the vinegar douche, mix one tablespoon of white vinegar with one gallon of water. The golden seal douche is made by steeping two bags of this tea in a pint of water, and cooling it before use. I usually recommend the golden seal douche because it creates a strong acid medium in the uterus, which helps prevent infections.

HEAD COLDS AND SINUS DRIP—Take a mustard footbath (see Influenza) twice a day to help break up congestion and relieve an acute sinus problem. In addition, double your intake of Vitamin C (according to your blood type) and drink rose-hip tea three times a day.

CHEST CONGESTION OR COUGHS—Treat these conditions as you would asthma. Reduce meat and dairy products according to your blood type. Type A's and AB's should follow a vegetarian regimen and B's and O's should temporarily go on a vegetarian/fish diet.

In addition, warm mustard footbaths and steam baths should be taken twice a day (see Influenza and Asthma) to disperse congestion. To also help break up mucus, shine a red light on your feet for fifteen minutes several times a day; this will stimulate the circulation in your feet and draw the blood downward from your chest, thus helping to discharge any concentrations in your lungs.

Another surefire remedy to ease congestion is a mixture of a tablespoon of the juice of one-half lemon, a tablespoon of honey and one tablespoon of brandy several times a day.

Kali. Sulph. is the suggested biochemic remedy when there is a cough with yellow expectorant, and Kali. Mur. if there is a white albuminous discharge.

HEMORRHOIDS—Hemorrhoids are caused by irregular bowel movements and undue strain put on the intestinal muscles during elimination. Blood is forced into the hemorrhoidal vein, which, over a period of time, distends and bulges. All blood types should eat more fruits and raw vegetables to promote the easy passage of wastes from the colon. Types O and B should reduce their intake of meat (which can have a constipating effect) and temporarily eat more fish.

When eliminating, try to make your bowel movements as complete as possible without straining. Remain on the toilet until you are certain no more wastes need to be eliminated. Often, after an incomplete evacuation acids can be secreted. These burn and itch your rectum, irritating the hemorrhoids. After a bowel movement, gently wash your rectum with lukewarm water and a mild soap, then pat the area with witch hazel.

INSOMNIA—Mental unrest is generally the cause of insomnia. The principal remedy is to learn to leave your problems on the night table upon retiring! Problems are never solved when you are tired and restless. Only with a clear and calm mind can you work through your difficulties.

Drinking a cup of a strong brew of chamomile or valerian-root tea before going to bed will help relax your nerves and promote a peaceful night's sleep. Increasing your calcium, pantothenic acid and B-complex vitamins will also have a soothing effect on your nervous system and help you to sleep.

SWOLLEN GLANDS—Lymph glands swell whenever infection is present or impurities are being filtered out of the body. I believe this swelling to be caused by wastes circulating in the bloodstream or by an open wound near a gland.

If your throat is swollen, gargle with a solution of vinegar and water or salt and water, or apply a poultice of clay and water (see Arthritis) or a boiled cabbage (see Sore Throat). These treatments will help to draw out the toxins and reduce the inflammation.

If your glands are swollen or infected in other parts of your

200

body, such as in the groin or under the armpits, you may apply a clay-and-water or a cold-water poultice.

In addition, focusing a green light on the inflamed area will promote healing, while increasing your Vitamin C intake (according to your blood type) will raise your body's resistance.

EARACHES—Hold a warm baked potato to your ear for fifteen minutes. Repeat several times a day until the inflammation has been drawn out and you no longer experience pain. Putting a drop or two of heated olive oil into your ear prior to applying the baked potato will also help to draw out the inflammation.

Another remedy is parboiling an onion (cut out the center core) and hold the onion directly against your ear. This, too, will relieve the inflammations and help reduce aches and ringing sensations. If pain persists or if there is a fever, consult your doctor.

GASTRIC DISTURBANCES—Most common gastric disturbances, such as flatulence, heartburn, acidity, stomach cramps and nausea, can be treated in a similar way: by improving your eating habits. I estimate that 75 percent of your gastric discomforts can be alleviated by combining or chewing your food properly, and by not speaking or drinking while you eat. Eating the more laxative foods—fruits and vegetables—before eating meat and grains, and taking a digestive enzyme tablet after each meal will further reduce these disorders.

To help soothe mild cramps or to reduce gas, drink chamomile or peppermint tea as needed. For severe cramps, drink golden seal tea or apply a cold-water poultice to your abdominal area for thirty minutes.

HALITOSIS—Bad breath is usually a reflection of an abdominal disorder. It can be brought on by bad eating habits, such as overeating or combining foods improperly, or from a highly acidic condition. The prime remedy for this problem is to correct your eating habits. However, the foul odor can temporarily be alleviated by chewing some parsley leaves or by taking chlorophyll or comfrey tablets.

DIARRHEA—Diarrhea is a symptom of many diseases and is an indication that the body is trying to eliminate unwanted matter. Among the many causes of diarrhea in adults are emotional upsets, eating unripe fruits and indigestible substances, food poisoning and catarrh in the stomach. Rest and warmth will give your body the chance to deal with the problem in its own way. Your diet should temporarily be restricted to binding foods, such as rye bread, concentrated blueberry juice (one tablespoon at a time), brown rice and baked potatoes. In addition, vegetables should be eaten steamed instead of raw to reduce the roughage in the intestines; and taking a combination of unflavored gelatin and apple peel will help to reduce loose stool.

Chamomile or golden seal tea has a healing effect on diarrhea induced by emotional upsets and should be drunk as often as desired.

Diarrhea is a common experience among people who travel and drink water in foreign countries. An opiated compound is often the medical prescription for such disorders. However, eating binding foods and taking Calc. Phos. will return the bowel movements to normal without the constipation that often follows treatment with the opiated drug.

COMMON HEADACHES—There are many causes of headaches, ranging from dietary disturbances to stress, poor eyesight, toothaches and sinus infections. Generally I have found a headache is caused by the accumulation of waste matter which creates pressure, depressions and throbbing. The best remedy, I believe, would be to give yourself an enema. High-protein food should be

202

temporarily avoided. A vegetarian or vegetarian/fish diet (according to your blood type) is preferable because proteins can increase toxicity, worsening the condition. A strong brew of chamomile tea is an excellent treatment for a throbbing head. A blue light creates a soothing environment, which is restful to the head.

Taking a cold footbath will also help to draw the toxic wastes from the stomach and thus reduce the problem. Immerse both feet in a tub or a basin of cold water for fifteen minutes as often as needed. A cold-water poultice can be used in lieu of the footbath with similar effect.

WORMS—Chewing and swallowing several cloves of garlic is, I have found, a highly effective remedy for worms in the intestines. If the case is severe, boil garlic in milk and drink this once or twice a day, or until the condition subsides. This remedy can also be used for your pets. If worms persist, see your doctor!

BOILS—Boils, like other skin disorders such as abscesses, pimples and acne, represent a retention of waste matter in the body. A proper dietary and detoxification program should be followed. In addition, increase your intake of Vitamin C and E (according to your blood type) to enhance capillary permeability and better circulation, which will promote tissue repair. To help purify your blood, drink red-clover tea three times a day. Golden seal tea may be drunk, in conjunction with, or infused into, a brew of red-clover to cleanse the blood.

PROSTATIC CONDITIONS—Although a complete treatment cannot be recommended for prostatic inflammations without a thorough diagnosis, you can begin to help yourself by eliminating spicy foods and meat products, which can be irritating to the prostate gland (uric acid in meat can be especially offensive to a tender and inflamed prostate gland).

203

Also, increase your Vitamin A intake to twice your daily dosage, and drink ten to twelve glasses of parsley water (steep a handful of parsley in hot water for ten minutes). I believe that parsley water will help heal an inflamed prostate and this brew can also be drunk by middle-aged men as a preventive measure.

SCIATICA—Sciatica is an inflammation of the sciatic nerve, which is felt at the back of the thigh. This can occur for a variety of reasons: exposure to dampness, or a chill, may irritate the nerve and a slipped disc can also cause sciatic pain. The effects can extend from the hip joint down to the foot, with the hips, knees and ankles becoming particularly tender. Frequently, an impaired sciatic nerve will inhibit mobility by making the movement of a limb exceedingly painful and thus confine one to bed.

A fern poultice can be a great relief to sciatic pressure and its accompanying pains. Boil female fern (obtainable in health food stores) lightly in water, soak a linen cloth in the infusion and apply to the lower back area along the sciatic nerve pathway.

A green light focused on the painful area and chamomile tea baths will also bring relief.

ANEMIA—Anemia is an impoverished condition of the blood, with either a deficiency of the red blood cells or the oxygen carrier, hemoglobin. This condition usually results from a deficient diet or from stress. It can also occur when there has been excessive bleeding after childbirth, or in other conditions when there is a considerable loss of blood.

If you are a type O, increase your consumption of calf's liver, veal and lamb for protein and iron. Types A and AB should increase their consumption of seeds, almonds, tofu and soy beans. B's should eat more fish and introduce veal and calf's liver into their diet once a week for protein and iron. All blood types can temporarily eat more eggs and should eat raisins as an iron source. Vegetables and fruits should be eaten in abundance to increase the vitamins and minerals in your body. Fresh air and sunshine will also be beneficial to patients with this condition.

B-complex vitamins should temporarily be increased to twice the daily dosage to fortify your body with protein. Ferrous iron tablets should also be temporarily increased to twice the daily dosage to promote red-blood-cell production. I am convinced that a disciplined exercise program is vital in treating this condition, for it will activate the blood, bring more oxygen into the body and thereby promote red-blood-cell proliferation.

Focusing a red light on your stomach for ten minutes every day will stimulate your body and also affect the production of new red blood cells.

HIGH CHOLESTEROL—As the fat, cholesterol, can accumulate in the arterial walls, your first step in reducing cholesterol in your blood is to reduce your consumption of animal products such as meats, cheese, eggs and fats. Reducing your starch and sugar intake is also crucial to controlling the condition: therefore, bread, grains and honey should be temporarily cut back.

To help purify your blood, drink red-clover tea three times a day. Mix lecithin granules in your salads and grains every day: the soy phosphatides in lecithin dissolve fats and resinous compounds in the arteries.

SPRAINS OR SORE MUSCLES—Steep a handful of linden tea in a pint of water, soak a linen cloth in the infusion and apply to the sore area for twenty minutes. A green light focused on the area for fifteen minutes a day will also promote healing.

CUTS, BURNS, ABRASIONS—Aloe vera gel is one of nature's best healing agents for minor wounds. A cut, burn or abrasion can quickly be healed by breaking a stem from an aloe vera plant and rubbing it on the wound, or by applying fresh aloe vera gel (available at health food stores) directly to the area. It can stop the formation of pus and infections, and hasten tissue repair.

Vitamin E oil is also an excellent curative and should be applied directly to the wound to encourage rapid healing.

MUSCLE OR JOINT ACHES—Massage peanut oil into the aching area as required. A green light focused on the area for fifteen minutes should also be used for relief.

INSECT BITES—Apply a leaf of stinging nettle plant directly to the bite. If this is unavailable, dig into the earth until you reach the red or yellow clay level and apply this to the bite area.

POISON IVY—Apply the leaf from the plant Impatiens to the irritations.

TOOTHACHES—Massage oil of cloves into the gum area as often as required. Crushed garlic may also be applied to the throbbing area.

CONSTIPATION—Constipation is the result of poor elimination, which causes the stool to become hard and dry within the colon. This can occur from the loss of flexibility in the intestinal muscles, or because the habit of regular bowel movements has not been developed.

An enema or herbal laxative will help flush the colon of wastes. Cold hip baths also have a stimulating effect on the bowels. For dietary suggestions see Chapter 10.

NERVOUS DISORDERS—Whenever emotional duress or undue mental stress exists, your nerves are robbed of their vitality.

In such cases, they must be brought back to a state of tranquility. Sitting in a room with a blue light for fifteen minutes every day will relax tension and stress. An occasional enema or fast (if your body is fit) will rid your body of acidity, which can stress the mind. Chamomile tea and warm baths are also recommended to relax and tone your nerves.

HEALTH VALUE OF HERBS

The following is a list of herbs and their uses. When using these for curative purposes, types O and B should make medium to strong infusions of the herbs; types A and AB should drink light or medium brews.

Name	Health Value
Bitter Aloe	Aids in stomach disorders.
Anise Seed	Makes a good eye lotion.
Arnica Flowers	Relieves stiffened, sore or painful joints.
Balm mint	Helps relieve abdominal troubles: gas, cramps and dyspepsia.
Barberries	Promotes healing of the liver and spleen.
Birch	Good for rheumatism, gout, dropsy.
Black-Adder-Tree Bark	A purgative.
Blackberry Leaves	A blood purifier.
Black Currant Leaves	Break up congestion of the chest.
Blackthorn Blossoms	Help strengthen the digestive system.
Blueberries	A good remedy for diarrhea.
Burdock Root	Stimulates the growth of hair.
Caraway	Relieves gas, cramps in the stomach and other general stomach complaints.
Chamomile	Relieves griping pains or cramps in the stomach; a calmative to the nerves.
Chickweed	Helps eliminate water from the body.
Chicory	Purifies the liver, kidneys and spleen.
Cloves (oil)	For toothaches.
Coltsfoot	Purifies the lungs.
Comfrey	A blood-purifier and nerve tonic.

Name	Health Value
Dandelion	A blood-purifier; also healing to the kidneys and bladder.
Elderberries	Aid in diarrhea and colic.
Eucalyptus	Promotes digestion.
Eyebright	An excellent cure for eye diseases.
Fennel	Helps relieve gas.
Fenugreek	Makes a good throat gargle, and poultice for drawing out swellings.
Fern	A purgative. Good for sciatic pain as a poultice.
Flaxseed	Helps draw out swellings and ulcers when used in a poultice.
Hayflower	Used for vapor baths and compresses.
Heather	Makes a good cough remedy; breaks up catarrh in throat and nose.
Hen's feet	Useful for jaundice, eruptions of the skin, piles.
Iceland Moss	Helps cure chest and lung troubles and general debility.
Juniper	Neutralizes foul breath; relieves flatulence; helps pass stones in the bladder.
Lavender	Relieves stomach problems and headaches.
Licorice	Excellent expectorant.
Linden Flowers	Help remove obstructions in the lungs; help bronchial disorders; when used in poultice helps sprains.
Liverwort	Helps stop hemorrhaging when directly applied; helps heal the liver.
Lungwort	Reduces catarrh in the lungs.
Marigold Flowers	Eliminate boils, ulcers, abscesses.
Marjoram	Excellent for irregular menstruation.
Mistletoe	Helpful in circulatory disturbances; when taken as a tea helps stop hemorrhages.
Mullein Flowers	Eliminate mucus in the chest.
Nettle	Breaks up mucus in the lungs.
Oats	Good for baths, packs and compresses.
Peppermint	Improves digestion
Periwinkle	Helps discharge mucus in intestines and lungs.
Primrose	Helpful in articular rheumatism.
Rhubarb	Good for stomach and intestinal troubles; a mild purgative.

208

Home Therapies

Name	Health Value
Ribwort	Loosens mucus in the inner organs.
Rosemary	Relieves stomach complaints.
St. Johns'wort	Disperses mucus in chest.
Sage	Useful for ailing liver and kidneys, and mucus in the throat and stomach.
Sandalwood	Stops the flow of blood in all kinds of hemorrhages.
Sarsaparilla	A blood-purifier.
Sassafras	Relieves asthma.
Shave-grass (common horsetail)	Used in compresses for sores containing pus. Cleans the stomach and alleviates the pain from stones in the bladder. Healing to the kidneys.
Shepherd's Purse	Stops hemorrhages of all kinds.
Strawberry Leaves	A blood-purifier. Very invigorating for convalescents.
Sweet Basil	Breaks up mucus obstructions in the lungs.
Thyme	Good for cramps in the stomach.
Valerian Root	Breaks up congestion in the head; calming to the nervous system.
Vervain	Soothing to cases of pains in the kidneys.
Violet	A splendid gargle for swollen throat.
Watercress	A blood-purifier.
Wormwood	A stomach remedy.

—Based on the teachings of Sebastian Kneipp

12

The Holistic Concept

Because my focus in this book has been on the nutritional aspects of natural healing, I have largely omitted discussing the effects the mind has on one's health. My intention has not been to imply that all there is to health is eating the right foods; rather, that the body has to be respected as a physical organism and that to function normally, without incurring physical breakdowns, it must receive a *specific* kind of nourishment.

But, nourishment is not restricted to food. People also require a diet of healthy thoughts. One of the great unanswerable questions that confounds all doctors is "Where does an illness really begin: in the body or in the mind?" For instance, does an ulcer occur because a person has eaten improperly? Or was it really caused by stress, fear or anxiety? Could these intangibles eat away at a person until there is a manifestation on the material plane of a bleeding abdominal sore?

One day, a woman came to my office complaining of insomnia and deep depressions. She was in her late twenties, but she looked at least fifteen years older: her face was haggard, her hair graying;

211

her body seemed lifeless. On examining her, I found no signs to account for her condition. Since I did not know her well, I couldn't figure out the nature of her distress, and therefore, put her on a general diet for her blood type.

During her first few visits she made no progress. It was apparent to me that she was severely disturbed by something, and I knew that her health would not improve until she overcame her emotional problem. I asked her if she wanted to talk to me about anything. She was shy and hesitant at first. I explained to her that I really couldn't help her unless she gave me a better idea of why she was so unhappy. Tearfully, she related the tale of how her best friend had stolen her fiancé, making her lose all hope of ever finding happiness again.

Her desperate state of mind had obviously infected every cell of her body: since she no longer cared about herself, her body had become worn, and prematurely aged. Only after our conversations week after week did she begin to realize that she had a whole life ahead of her; that she could be a fruitful and productive person, and fall in love again. As she gained a more optimistic outlook, her deadened body slowly revived to become as vibrant and alive as her new attitude.

The mind is a powerful tool. Sometimes it is a weapon that, too often, people use against themselves. "As a man thinketh, so he is." While diet is fundamental to the body's physical well-being, clear, positive thinking must exist concomitantly, keeping one's spirits high and one's will strong enough to meet the challenges of daily living.

Many people believe that all you have to do is eat properly and your life will automatically fall into place. Others argue that the mind completely controls the biochemic reactions occurring simultaneously in the body, such as the digestion of food, the circulation of oxygen, the creation and destruction of cells, and consequently their health. But, neither body nor mind is one hundred percent responsible for health.

It's impossible to estimate the exact balance of body and mind that determines one's health. For argument's sake, let's say that the mind is 45 percent responsible for a person's well-being and the physical body, 55 percent. If your body is improperly nourished, your organs are robbed of their physiological vitality, hence, your body's systems will not function effectively. A reduction of physical vitality has a corresponding effect on mental clarity, happiness and inward tranquility. Consequently, your mind's control over your body is diminished to maybe 40 or 30 percent. Because your mind is no longer working efficiently, both body and mind will experience a spiraling decrease in their ability to work properly.

As Dr. Hahnemann said, a person is a "rounded whole." The body must be fed or both it and the mind will suffer. The mind has to be positive and strong or both mind and body will be adversely affected.

The body and mind are major parts of the whole human system. Neither has been fully understood. However, each must be respected for its contribution to the makeup of the individual, and each must be nourished.

This is the basis of the holistic concept of health care I mentioned in the opening pages of this book. My many years' experience in helping countless patients has convinced me that the holistic approach is the surefire way in which to help people lead healthy, productive and fulfilled lives.

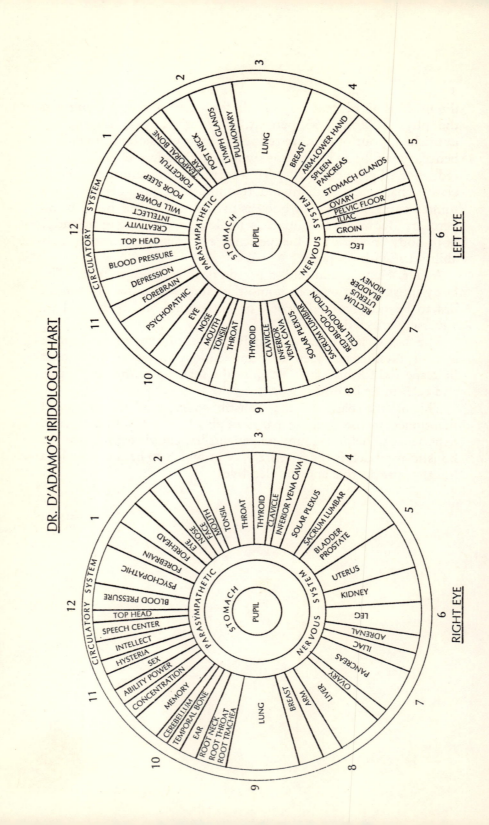

DR. D'ADAMO'S IRIDOLOGY CHART

SIGNS IN THE EYES

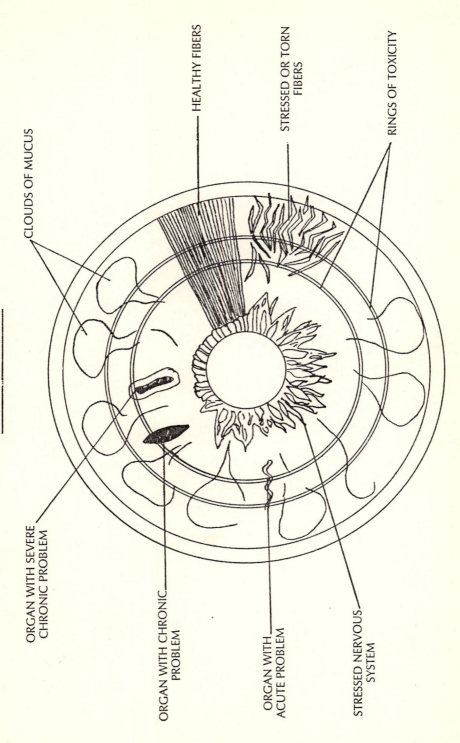

CLOUDS OF MUCUS

HEALTHY FIBERS

STRESSED OR TORN FIBERS

RINGS OF TOXICITY

ORGAN WITH SEVERE CHRONIC PROBLEM

ORGAN WITH CHRONIC PROBLEM

ORGAN WITH ACUTE PROBLEM

STRESSED NERVOUS SYSTEM

Bibliography and Recommended Readings

Aichele, Ditmar, and Renate Aichele, and Heinze Schwegler and Anneliese Schwegler: *Der KosmosPflanzenfurer*, W. Keller and Co., Stuttgart, 1978.

Alvarez, W.: *An Introduction to Gastroenterology*, Paul Hoeber, Inc., New York, 1948.

Babkin, B. P.: *Secretory Mechanism of Digestive Glands*, Paul Hoeber, Inc., New York, 1950.

Bach, Edward: *Heal Thyself (An Explanation of the Real Cause and Cure of Disease)*, C. W. Daniel Co., Ltd., England, 1931.

Blackie, Margery G.: *The Patient, Not the Cure*, MacDonald and James, London, 1976.

Boericke, William: *A Compendium of the Principles of Homeopathy as Taught by Hahnemann*, Health Research, California, 1896.

Cannon, W. B.: *The Mechanical Factors of Digestion*, Longmans, Greene and Co., Ltd., London, 1911.

Carson, Rachel: *Silent Spring*, Houghton Mifflin, Boston, 1962.

Challoner, H. K.: *The Path of Healing,* The Theosophical Publishing House, London, 1972.

Copen, Bruce: *A Rainbow of Health,* Academic Publications, England, 1974.

————: *Heal Yourself with Colour,* Academic Publications, England, 1950.

Coulter, Harris, L.: *Homeopathic Medicine,* Formur, Inc., St. Louis, 1972.

Culpeper, Nicholas: *The Complete Herbal and English Physician,* Reprinted in Great Britain by A. Wheaton & Co., Exeter. Copyright W. Favisham & Co., Ltd.

Dane, Victor: *Colors and Their Effects on Health,* California, 1956.

Davenport, H. W.: *Physiology of the Digestive Tract,* Year Book Medical Publishers, Chicago, 1961, 1966.

Davidson, Victor S.: *Science of Iris Diagnosis,* Essence of Health, South Africa, 1970.

Dufty, Willia: *Sugar Blues,* Chilton, Radnor, Pennsylvania, 1975.

Eaves, A. Osborne: *The Color Cure,* California, 1956.

Fredericks, Carlton, and Herman Goodman: *Low Blood Sugar and You,* Grosset and Dunlap, New York, 1969.

Freund, Leopold: *Elements of General Radio-Therapy,* London Publications, London, 1904.

Ganzfried, Solomon: *Code of Jewish Law,* Hebrew Publishing Co., New York, 1961.

Garten, M. O.: *The Health Secrets of a Naturopathic Doctor,* Parker Publishing Co., Inc., New York, 1967.

Goodman, Louis S., and Alfred Gilman (ed.).: *The Pharmacological Basis of Therapeutics, Fifth Edition,* Macmillan, New York, 1975.

Guyton, A. C.: *Textbook of Medical Physiology,* W. B. Saunders Co., Philadelphia, 1961.

Hahnemann, Samuel: *The Chronic Diseases (Their Peculiar Nature and Their Homeopathic Cure),* Jain Publishing Co., New Delhi, 1975.

Heline, Corinne: *Healing and Regeneration Through Color,* California, 1956.

218

Hewlett-Parsons, J. D.: *The ABC's of Nature Cures,* Arco Publishers Co., New York, 1968.

Holmes, Ernest: *The Science of the Mind,* Dodd, Mead and Co., New York, 1938.

Howat, R. Douglas: *Elements of Chromotherapy,* The Actinic Press, Ltd., London, 1938.

Huxley, Aldous: *Perennial Philosophy,* Chatto and Windus, London, 1969.

Kellogg, J. H.: *The Itinerary of a Breakfast,* Funk and Wagnalls Co., New York, 1926.

Kriege, Theodor: *Fundamental Basis of Iris Diagnosis.* L. N. Fowler and Co., Ltd., London, 1975.

Kuenzle, John: *Herbs and Weeds,* Health Research, California.

Kuhne, Louis: *The New Science of Healing,* Health Research, California.

Lewis, Alvin E.: *Principles of Hematology,* Appleton-Century-Crofts, New York, 1970.

Luyties, F. August: *The Biochemic Handbook,* Formur, Inc., St. Louis, 1970.

Muntner, Suessman: *Moses Maimonides,* 2 vols., Bloch Publishing Co., 1970.

Nielsen, Harold: *Heilpflanzen in Farbe,* BLV Verslagsgesellschaf, Munich, 1977.

Null, Gary and Steve Null: *The Complete Handbook of Nutrition,* Robert Speller & Sons, New York, 1972.

Palmer, D. D.: *The Chiropractor,* Health Research, Mokelumne Hill, California, 1914.

Pavlov, I. P.: *The Work of the Digestive Glands,* C. Griffin Co., London, 1902.

Rapaport, Samuel I.: *Introduction to Hematology,* Harper & Row, New York, 1971.

Rolf, Ida P.: *Rolfing,* Dennis-Landman Publishers, California, 1977.

Ross, A. C. Gordon: *Homeopathy (An Introductory Guide).* England, 1976.

Schomburg, Eberhard: *Sebastian Kneipp,* Sanitas Verlag, K.G., Bad Worishofen, 1963.

Shears, Curtis C.: *Health Education,* Gloucestershire, England: Castle Press, Berkeley, 1974.

Shelton, Herbert M.: *Food Combining Made Easy,* Dr. Shelton's Health School, San Antonio, 1951.

———: *Health for the Millions,* Natural Hygiene Press, Inc., Chicago, 1968.

Smith, H.: *The Molecular Biology of Plant Cells,* University of California Press, Berkeley and Los Angeles, 1977.

Spangler, David: *The Laws of Manifestation,* Findhorn Publications, Scotland, 1976.

Starr-White, George: *Color Healing,* California, 1956.

Swami Budhananda: *The Mind and Its Control,* Venda Press, Hollywood, 1974.

Swami Prabhavananda (tr.): *Bhagavad-Gītā,* The American Library, New York, 1944.

Tilden, J. H.: *Impaired Health, Its Cause and Cure,* (new printing), Health Research, Mokelumne Hill, California, 1959.

Tobe, John H.: *Proven Herbal Remedies,* Provoker Press, Canada, 1969.

Todd, Mabel Elsworth: *The Thinking Body,* Paul Hoeber, Inc., New York, 1937.

Verner, J. R., C.W. Weiant, and R. J. Watkins: *Rational Bacteriology,* H. Wolff, New York, 1953.

Vida-Deck: *Klinische Prufung der Organ-und Krankheitszeichen in der Iris,* 1954.

Weir, John, and Margaret L. Tyler: *Homeopathic Drug Pictures.*

Wendel, Paul: *The Basic Teachings of Father Sebastian Kneipp.* Self-Published, Brooklyn, 1947.

Winter, Ruth: *A Consumer's Dictionary of Cosmetic Ingredients,* Crown Publishers, New York, 1976.

Wren, R. C.: *Potter's New Cyclopedia of Botanical Drugs and Preparations,* Health Science Press, England, 1973.

Yesudian, Selvarajan, and Elizabeth Haich: *Yoga and Health,* Harper & Row, New York, 1953.

Index

Index

diet for arthritic, 86–87
health care program for, 75–79
individualized diet for, 98–100
type O-blood individuals compared
  with, 47–48
vitamin/mineral program for, 42, 44,
  127, 129–34
weight-reduction program for, 61–62
Type AB-blood individuals, 33–34, 36
diet for, in balanced state of health,
  50–53, 58–59
diet for arthritic, 88
health care program for, 83–85
individualized diet for, 98, 100, 115–
  18
type AB-blood individuals compared
  with, 51–53
vitamin/mineral program for, 52,
  144–47
weight-reduction program for, 61–62
Type B-blood individuals, 33–37
diet for, in balanced state of health,
  47–51, 56–58
diet for arthritic, 87–88
health care program for, 81–83
individualized diet for, 99, 101, 110–15
type AB-blood individuals compared
  with, 52
type O-blood individuals compared
  with, 50
vitamin/mineral program for, 50,
  139–44
weight-reduction program for, 65–66
Type O-blood individuals, 33–37
diet for, in balanced state of health,
  44–47, 55–56
diet for arthritic, 86–87
individualized diet for, 98–101, 108–10
type AB-blood individuals compared
  with, 52, 53
type B-blood individuals compared
  with, 48
vitamin/mineral program for, 47, 127,
  134–38
weight-reduction program for, 63–64

Veal, *see* Meats and poultry
Vegetables and fruits, 12, 29, 30, 31
arthritis and, 193
digestion of, 162–63, 174, 175
after fasting, 184
health value of, 118–23

in home remedies, 198, 200–2, 204–5
organic, 70
pesticides on, 69
in promotion of bowel movements, 181
for type A-blood individuals, 34, 40–41,
  43–44, 54–55, 75–78, 104–6
for type AB-blood individuals, 51–52,
  58–59, 83–84, 116–18
for type B-blood individuals, 48, 49, 57,
  81, 83, 111–15
for type O-blood individuals, 45–47,
  55–56, 79, 80, 109
vibrational level of, 37
waiting period when fruit is eaten
  before meal, 62, 64, 66
Violet (color), therapy with, 191
Vitamin A, 71, 127, 155, 194, 204
for type A-blood individuals, 44, 130,
  133, 134
for type AB-blood individuals, 144, 146
for type B-blood individuals, 50, 139,
  141–43
for type O-blood individuals, 135, 137,
  138
Vitamin B-complex, 60, 127, 196, 200
pantothenic acid for type O-blood individuals, 135
primary sources of, 155
  for type A-blood individuals, 44, 129,
    130, 133, 134
  for type AB-blood individuals, 144, 146
  for type B-blood individuals, 50, 139–43
  for type O-blood individuals, 47, 135,
    137, 138
in whole-wheat products, 71
Vitamin C, 12, 127, 156
effects of smoking on, 104, 135, 145
in home remedies, 194–96, 199, 201,
  203
for type A-blood individuals, 130–31,
  133, 134
for type AB-blood individuals, 144–47
for type B-blood individuals, 139,
  141–43
for type O-blood individuals, 135, 137
Vitamin D, 127, 156
for type A-blood individuals, 130, 134
for type AB-blood individuals, 144, 146
for type B-blood individuals, 139,
  141–43
for type O-blood individuals, 50, 135,
  137, 138

Vitamin E, 127, 156, 203, 206
  for type A-blood individuals, 44, 130,
    131, 134
  for type AB-blood individuals, 144, 146
  for type B-blood individuals, 139,
    141–43
  for type O-blood individuals, 135, 137,
    138
Vitamin K, 156
Vitamin M (folic acid), 157
Vitamin P (bioflavonoid), 157
Vitamin/mineral program, 20, 24–25,
  125–27
  and effects of alcohol on vitamins, 72
  and mineral value of herbs, 149–54
  for type A-blood individuals, 42, 44,
    127, 129–34
  for type AB-blood individuals, 52,
    144–47
  for type B-blood individuals, 49, 139–44
  for type O-blood individuals, 47, 127,
    134–38

vital minerals listed, 148–49
and vitamin values of foods, 155–57
See also specific vitamins and minerals

Water, 12, 71, 89
Weight-reduction program, 60–66
Whole-wheat products, 71, 174
  for type A-blood individuals, 105, 106
  for type AB-blood individuals, 51, 116,
    117
  for type B-blood individuals, 57, 112,
    113, 115
  for type O-blood individuals, 45, 55,
    109
Worms, home remedy for, 203

Yeast, 132
Yellow (color), therapy with, 189–90

Zinc, 131, 148